SLAYING

the

DRAGON

Treating Alcohol and Drug Related Illnesses With Chinese Herbs

THOMAS R. JOINER

Books by Thomas Richard Joiner

Blending Botany with Budo

Chinese Herbal Medicine Made Easy

Kung Fu Medicine

Martial Esoterica

Slaying the Dragon

The Warrior as Healer

SLAYING
the
DRAGON

Treating Alcohol and Drug Related Illnesses With Chinese Herbs

SEA OF CHI PUBLISHING
OAKLAND, CA

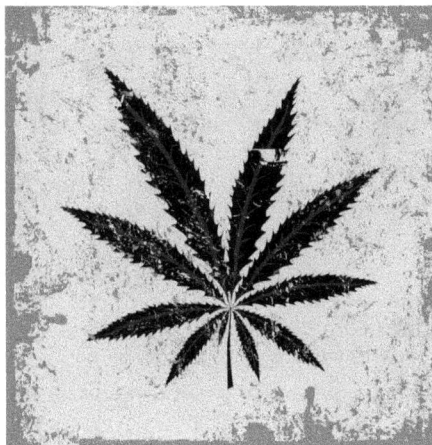

SEAOFCHI.COM
Seaofchi.com Publishing
200 Montecito Avenue # 304
Oakland, CA 94610
1-800-641-0945
1-510-451-0945
info@seaofchi.com

Note to reader: This book is intended as an information guide. The remedies, approaches, and techniques described herein are meant to supplement, and not to be a substitute for, professional medical care or treatment. They should not be used to treat a serious ailment without prior consultation with a qualified health care professional.

Library of Congress Cataloging-in-Publication Data
Joiner, Thomas Richard, 1943-
Slaying the Dragon: Treating alcohol and drug related illnesses with Chinese herbs/ Thomas Richard Joiner._1st ed.p. cm. Includes biographical references and index. ISBN: 9780615881928 (alk. Paper) 1. Herbs-Therapeutic use. 2. Addiction-Alternative treatment. 3. Medicine, Chinese. I. Title.
Library of Congress Control Number: 1-1007836483.
Registration Number: TXu 1-886-116.

Printed and bound in USA.
Manufactured in the USA.
10 9 8 7 6 5 4 3 2 1

Editor: Jennifer Grace, expertsubjects.com
Cover Designer: Zoe Shtorm, zoeshtorm.com
Interior Designer: Catherine Murray, expertsubjects.com
Indexes: Judy Joiner

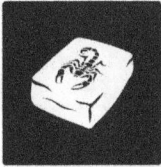

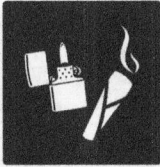

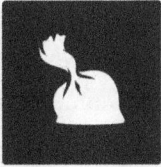

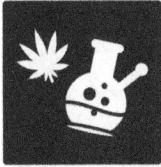

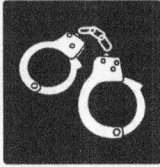

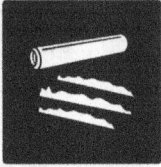

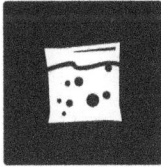

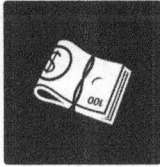

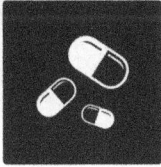

Contents

Dedication

A Family Affair

For most of us childhood memories are a flash-back to some of the happiest times of our lives. Who could forget those fairy-tale years? Odds are it was probably reflections on the pleasures of that tender age that inspired the adage: remembrance of adolescence never fails to warm the heart, because it's the summer of our youth that's the source of some of our most cherished memories. Regrettably, that's not always true.

Make no mistake we definitely had our share of laughs, but along with the good times there were also times when we laughed until our sides ached always mindful that in the blink of an eye fun and laughter could give way to an alcohol-driven rage. Like the pause in a storm when a transient ray of sunlight allows birds to briefly leave their shelter and chatter among themselves, family reunions were just a temporary diversion from the turbulence that was always festering beneath the surface.

Even though I always suspected that we were slightly dysfunctional, it was during one of those family gatherings of the worst kind that my suspicions were confirmed. That's when I first noticed, with the exception of my great-aunt Ellen, who was a dyed-in-the-wool Christian; all of my other family members who never agreed on anything did have two things in common. They all drank alcohol, and more importantly they drank it on a daily basis. Even though there were the usual telltale signs the full extent of alcohol's influence on our lives didn't register until the day that Grandma affectionately known as "Big Mama," departed for her final rest.

With wounded hearts we struggled to come to terms with the fact that our beloved Queen mother was gone. As we sat there defenseless against an onslaught of inconsolable grief, as my uncle Bennie often said, "The silence was so intense you could hear a gnat pissing on cotton."

Other than the occasional outburst of wailing and moaning that briefly erupted on the ride home from the cemetery, not a word was spoken. Spellbound, we all sat with our eyes glazed over; desperately searching for anything that could relieve the unbearable heartache that left us staring aimlessly with a faraway look in our eyes. We remained in that semi-catatonic state until quite unexpectedly the silence was shattered by the sizzling sound of a pot boiling over.

Startled by the unsolicited intrusion, we struggled to gather our wits as we went in search of the cause of the commotion. The closer we got to the source of the sizzle, the stronger the aroma of fried chicken became, as we made our way down the hall to the kitchen. Carefully avoiding the chair where Big Mama usually sat, I took a seat at the kitchen table and immediately began working on a strategy to try to convince Mom to let me have one of the drumsticks.

As I sat there thinking about the first mouthwatering bite, suddenly it occurred to me that everything else would have to wait because there was only one thing that was capable of constraining the gut-wrenching despair that could erupt at any moment into a full-blown emotional outbreak. Removing her apron, Mom placed a fifth of Johnny Walker Scotch in the center of the table and handed each adult a glass. As the bottle passed from one person to the next, each one filled his/her glass to the rim and hurriedly drank the contents. Returning their empty glasses to the table, there was a noticeable reaction to the jolt caused by the alcohol hitting their systems. Slowly… the Johnny Walker began taking effect. It was at that moment that it finally dawned on me that it really didn't matter whether we were celebrating life mourning death or simply gathering to break bread and re-establish family ties, alcohol was an established necessity getting them through both good and bad times.

Like a light bulb that's turned on in a darkened room revealing previously unseen things, suddenly I realized that despite their best effort they were incapable of overriding the genetic pre-programming that was like a family curse handed down one generation to the next from mother to daughter and father to son. An essential nutrient—alcohol—was life sustaining, it was their water of life.

In the years that followed an unfortunate result of their seemingly unquenchable thirst was the noticeable increase in requiem gatherings that began occurring as alcohol-related diseases started taking their toll, and like a chain reaction one family member after another was stricken.

Although through the grace of God, a few were spared the usual pain and suffering. Regrettably, it was alcohol-related diseases that claimed the lives of nearly all of the aunts, uncles, and cousins who sat at the kitchen table and drank a toast celebrating Big Mama's arrival at the pearly gates. On what will always be remembered as one of the saddest days of my life.

Slaying the Dragon was written for family members and friends who lived life on their own terms, and in spite of often being under the influence, showed me tough unconditional love during the best and worst of times. This book is dedicated to all of you and last but not least, to my wife Judy Joiner and my mother Ruby Blanchard (10/22/24-1/21/82)… R.I.P. Mom.

In Memorium

Joyce Elaine Joiner Otis Smith…Sis
Bennie Belcher Jr…Uncle Bennie
Mackinley Belcher…Uncle Mac
Gilbert Muckle…Muk-Muk
Dwight Otis…Baby Boy
Tomie Joiner…Daddy
Harvey and Sparrow
Ethel and Neal
James Moore
Lou Waters

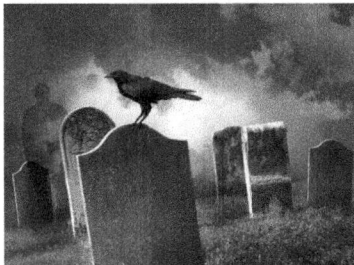

About the Author

It was one of those beautiful spring days when the air's filled with avian sounds and the senses are treated to the delectable fragrance of blossoms on a gentle breeze. That's when a casual stroll through New York's Thompkins Square Park was interrupted when I paused to watch a martial artist perform the classic kung fu form known as Eighteen Buddha Hand. In hind-sight I doubt that anyone could have predicted how much my life would be changed by that chance encounter, not even someone with psychic abilities.

After observing the breathtaking execution of the quintessential kung fu form not only did it inspire me to begin training in the martial arts, it also ultimately led to my discovery of Chinese herbal medicine which became my life's work. Over the years I've come to realize that the events that took place that day were undoubtedly a result of astral influences that were advanced by that inexplicable introduction to the fighting arts.

Since that life changing encounter more than thirty years ago, I've trained in what I believe is one of martial art's preeminent styles and advanced to the level of Kyoshi 6th Dan in the Chinese Goju System. I had the honor of receiving the University of Martial Arts and Science Humanitarian Award for Notable Achievement and Excellence in Holistic Medicine; I was inducted into the Chinese Goju Hall of Fame by Grandmaster Shidoshi Ron Van Clief in 1994, and became a member of Chinese Goju International in 2013.

My background in Chinese medicine/Herbology includes: clinical internship in Chinese Medicine (Acupuncture) that was part of a three-and-a-half-year work/study program at the Institute of Traditional Chinese Medicine First World Acupuncture New York City, advanced acupuncture and Chinese Herbology under Dr. Lai Fu Cai at the Academy of Chinese Culture and Health Sciences in Oakland, CA., and Chinese

Herbology at the Institute of Chinese Herbology Berkeley, CA. I have also done an extensive study of Tien Tao Chi Kung, and Taoist, Christian, and Rosicrucian philosophies, as well as being the founder and president of an on-line company Treasures from the Sea of Chi that sells Chinese herbs for general health, and specializes in herbs used in martial arts training.

I've written six books: *The Warrior as Healer, Chinese Herbal Medicine Made Easy, Blending Botany and Budo, Martial Esoterica, Kung Fu Medicine,* and most recently *Slaying the Dragon,* in addition to being a contributing editor for Martialforce.com a martial arts e-magazine.

That said, I should mention that a guiding principle in all aspects of my life is my belief that there are no coincidences. Every event in our lives is a result of (universal, cosmic, karmic) law which ultimately determines our destiny and everything that happens… happens for a reason!

My life journey has brought me to this place in time for the singular purpose of writing this book. The idea for writing the book which I have given the implausible title *Slaying the Dragon,* is a result of years of training in traditional Chinese medicine/ Herbology, as well as drawing upon childhood memories of growing up watching neighbors, friends, and family members in an on-going struggle with health issues that were often a direct result of poverty and substance abuse.

As fate would have it, an introduction to acupuncture and Chinese Herbology that was part of my early Wing Chun kung fu training, turned out to be the perfect vehicle in my search for a way to help poor, medically underserved, mostly minority communities, deal with some of the problems associated with substance abuse and addiction.

The five-thousand-year-old medicine's use of natural ingredients, its proven curative capability, its ability to treat practically every disease known to man and the fact that Chinese herbs can be used effectively by someone with little or no medical training are just a few of the reasons I was drawn to the centuries-old healing art.

Another influencing factor in my decision to study the ancient medicine, was Chinese medicine's well-documented history of successfully treating drug abuse and dependency (namely opium addiction) which I believe makes it uniquely qualified for treating illnesses associated with alcohol and drugs.

As in all of my previous books my primary goal in writing *Slaying the Dragon* is to empower people with health-management skills by providing insights into traditional Chinese medicine, as well as furnishing herbal prescriptions that give them the ability to use herbs to effectively treat ailments like those described in chapter three of this book.

In addition to the book's main goal of providing information about how Chinese herbs can be used to treat alcohol and drug related illness, *Slaying the Dragon* is also an honorarium that was written for all of our departed loved ones who were lost along the way to alcohol and drugs.

Introduction

Even though in the U.S. there's far greater access to alternative forms of medical treatment than in years past, I still shutter whenever I think about the days when anyone stricken with an illness that castor oil or aspirin was incapable of curing only had two options -- prescription drugs, or worse the dreaded scalpel. If the current level of interest in alternative medicine is any indication, it's apparent that I'm not the only one who found the limited treatment options unsettling. Unlike in years past when interest in treatments other than conventional Western medicine was minimal at best, nowadays when people discover that I'm into Chinese herbs, I'm usually besieged with a million and one questions about the ancient healing art.

With consumer dissatisfaction at an all-time high, there seems to be no end to the growing list of complaints about the American health-care system. Although there is displeasure over a wide range of issues, most critics agree that when you narrow it down, the three main reasons for the rise in interest in alternative medicine are a desire to avoid surgery, the sky-rocketing cost of Western medical treatment, and concern over the negative side effects of pharmaceutical drugs.

While there's no question that fear of going under the knife, and living in a drugged state in order to remain pain-free are definitely cause for concern, for the average working-class American, perhaps the greatest fear is reaching the point where he/she can no longer afford medical care. Sadly, in recent years the escalating cost of health care has become so expensive that it's forcing all except the wealthy to try and fend off illness while they frantically search for an affordable alternative. Despite the creation of Obamacare and questionable reforms in the American health care system, unacceptable numbers of people continue to fall through the cracks when it comes to affordable healthcare. Many of these average and lower-income earners, who may or may not have health insurance, usually fall into one of two categories. Those who know absolutely nothing about Chinese Herbology, and those who have heard of it but due to cultural differences mainly centering on language, have been stymied in their attempt to learn more about the five-thousand-year-old healing art. As you can imagine the first thing that people want to know when you get into a discussion about Chinese herbs is are they effective, or do they work? After informing them that herbs are capable of treating everything from the common cold to cancer, normally the next topic of conversation involves correcting some important misinformation about some of the substances used in the ancient herbal system.

When you consider that for the average person the term "herbs" conjures up images of botanical substances such as: mushrooms, flowers, bark, roots, and twigs etc. that are used to treat illness. It's understandable why many of them are shocked when I inform them that Chinese Herbology also uses things like minerals, insects, and animal parts.

Like most newcomers, when I first learned about some of the weird substances used in the ancient medicine there was absolutely no way to convince me that anyone who was willing to ingest these questionable ingredients had not taken leave of their senses!

Not in my wildest imaginings did I suspect that in time, not only would I overcome my aversion to some of the substances used in the ancient herbal system. In the end I would also be helping others to come to terms with their misgivings about these strange medicinal items. Even though I still find some of these "exotic ingredients" and their seemingly inexplicable ability to cure disease a little odd, I'm convinced when it comes to drug-free therapies for treating practically every disease known to man there's no question Chinese Herbology is one of the world's most effective forms of alternative medicine.

Now I'd be the first to admit the idea of using bugs and animal parts that you're not likely to find at your local butcher shop to treat illness can be a stretch for most people. In fact, its concerns over some of the ancient medicine's strange ingredients that is often the determining factor when it comes to getting the average person beyond curious conversation to the actual practice of using herbs.

If you're wondering why I make such a big deal about trying to turn people on to Chinese herbs my honest answer, is after witnessing the healing power of herbs during my internship, not only did it help to resolve any lingering doubts about its effectiveness, it also convinced me that more than simple folk medicine Chinese Herbology is a sacred art that has never received the respect it deserves for its important role throughout history in minimizing the suffering of mankind.

I believe that when you teach people how to use nature's divine gift, it provides them with an alternative to the undesirable and sometimes dangerous side-effects of Western pharmaceutical medicine. This valuable health maintenance skill can contribute to better health and in some cases relieve un-necessary pain and suffering. When you compare the cost of herbs to high priced prescription drugs, possessing basic herbal skills provides an affordable option. This cost differential is especially important for people living on the poverty level who can't afford the high cost of Western medical treatment and far too often suffer in silence.

Years of working in acupuncture clinics, at the Institute of Traditional Chinese Medicine in New York City and Oakland's Academy of Chinese Culture and Health Sciences as part of my internship in traditional Chinese medicine, gave me the opportunity to observe first-hand the ancient medicine's effectiveness in treating common illnesses, as well as ailments that are often a result of life-styles that include alcohol and/or drug use. Those early observations of acupuncture and Chinese herbal medicine's effectiveness in treating illnesses associated with the two inebriants, was the inspiration for writing this book.

Ancient Cures for Modern Ills

Despite the fact that a recent study conservatively estimates that nearly thirty-five to forty percent of the population in the U.S. has been treated with acupuncture, Chinese herbs, or both, a surprising number of Americans are unaware that not only is the ancient medicine capable of treating everything from simple headaches to life-threatening internal diseases, but there is also ample clinical evidence that substantiates its effectiveness in treating illnesses associated with the different forms of substance abuse.

Although it's one of the least-publicized abilities of the ancient healing art, references to traditional Chinese medicine's role in treating alcohol and drug-related illnesses including withdrawal and detoxification, has been written about in modern medical literature as well as in some of China's oldest texts dating back thousands of years.

In the spirit of the ancient texts, *Slaying the Dragon* was written to help people who prefer using natural remedies how to use Chinese herbs, to treat health issues that can develop from too much drinking and drugging. Whether I succeed or not will depend on whether those who suffer from alcohol or drug-related illnesses are able to use the herbal formulas in the book to effectively treat them, as well as my ability to promote public understanding that addiction is a disease whose solution lies in decriminalization and treatment.

The People's Medicine...
Prescriptions from the Land of the Dragon

By most estimates it was fifty centuries ago give or take a few years that traditional Chinese medicine developed from seeds planted long before there was industry, agricultural systems, or organized states. Many medical scholars claim that the ancient healing art, which is only pre-dated by India's Ayurvedic tradition, can be traced all the way back to pre-historic times when the primary health care providers were shaman, witch doctors, sages, lamas and medicine men.

The treatment methods of these primordial physicians grew out of tribal healing practices that involved the use of charms, ritual magic and incantations. There was also a shared belief among these ancient healers that all illness was a result of malevolent spirits or demons that had taken possession of the body, and the only way to affect a cure and restore someone's health was by exorcising or casting them out. According to ancient belief, the way to accomplish this was with ritual drumming, that created hypnotic entrancing rhythms, and by casting spells and administering potions that were empowered by intoning sacred words. Today's modern traditional Chinese medicine is a result of human experiments, intellectual growth, and scientific advancement that spans the ages and is deeply rooted in the ancient healing practices that can be traced all the way back to these early beginnings.

Out of the different therapies that make up the traditional Chinese medical system (acupuncture, herbal medicine, food therapy, moxabustion, plum blossom, cupping, Tui Na (massage) etc.), in no other therapy are the overtones of primitive healing practices more apparent than in the practice of herbal medicine. The use of ingredients like snakeskin, animal bone, and roots and stones, appears to be a throw-back to practices from centuries past when it is likely that in addition to their medicinal use, these items were also associated with mystical practices like divination and ceremonial magic. While there's no disputing that the passing of time and advances in science have brought about dramatic changes, many of the core concepts of the ancient medicine, such as the belief that man's relationship with nature and the environment has a profound influence on one's health, continues to be one of its most important guiding principles. For some it's the combining of ancient theories and modern science that gives Chinese medicine its appeal. While for others, the fact that some of its principles and theories are not supported by Western scientific research often unjustifiably casts doubt on its efficacy.

Be that as it may it's safe to say that there are some similarities shared by traditional Chinese medicine and its Western counterpart, as well as some significant differences. One of the most important characteristics that underscore the contrasting views of the two medicines is that unlike Western pharmaceutical medicine, since its creation nearly five-thousand-years-ago, Chinese herbal medicine has remained in the hands of the Chinese people. Unlike Western prescription drugs, Chinese herbs are not controlled by a government drug commission, doctors, pharmaceutical companies or pharmacists. Throughout China's history since the-curative-ability of medicinal plants was first discovered, herbs have always been accessible to anyone in need of them.

Today, as in years past, herbs are readily available and can be purchased in herb stores for treating minor ailments as well as serious life-threatening diseases. This unrestricted public access is in stark contrast to Western medicine's requirement to visit a state-licensed doctor's office in order to obtain a prescription for high-priced pharmaceutical drugs for everything except over-the-counter medicine for treating minor illnesses.

And while most would agree that having access to medicine is important, some might argue that an even more compelling feature that distinguishes one medicine from the other is traditional Chinese medicine's emphasis on identifying the underlying cause for a particular illness rather than simply treating the illness's physical symptoms.

When people are first introduced to traditional Chinese medicine they're often surprised at the amount of scrutiny given to evaluating a patient's emotional/spiritual well-being, and the importance in bringing these elements into balance along with resolving any physical complaints as part of the over-all treatment. This "body, mind, spirit" approach to treatment which has unquestionable value in regard to health in general, has even greater significance when it comes to treating substance abuse based on sociological studies that have determined beyond physical dependency, psychological and/or spiritual matters are at the root of all of the different forms of substance abuse and addiction.

Other dissimilarities between the two medicines are Chinese herbal medicine's relatively low cost when compared to high-priced prescription drugs and their lack of negative side-effects and overall safety compared to Western chemical medicines. More significantly, herbs can be administered with a minimal amount of training. It is in fact, the effectiveness of herbs in the hands of those who lack technical training that is the main reason for herbal medicine's popularity and continued use for thousands of years by Taoist sages and master herbalists, as well as ordinary people who possess little or no formal medical training. This long-acknowledged, user-friendly nature has made it possible for novices to effectively use

Chinese herbs for treating illnesses such as those described in this book.

Over the years I have learned that through a conscious effort to use simple language and avoid complex medical terms, I have been able to get people who lack medical training to understand some of the basic principles of Chinese medicine, which has enabled them to effectively incorporate herbs into their daily lives to maintain their health. Although there are a few precautions that need to be taken into consideration when using Chinese herbs, such as not combining certain ingredients known to be antagonistic when used together. With few exceptions when the correct amount of each ingredient is used in a formula's preparation and the recommended dosage is strictly followed, most Chinese herbal formulas can be safely administered by someone with little or no experience.

That said, it would be irresponsible not to mention that in all cases of illness diagnosis by a skilled physician is highly recommended. If any doubt exists about the first diagnosis a second opinion should be sought. Once you receive a definitive diagnosis, if you make the decision to treat the condition with Chinese herbs this information should be shared with your regular doctor/primary physician (if you have one). Some will take a positive attitude, others will prefer to wait and see, and some may be less than encouraging. In any event, it should not be forgotten that making choices concerning the type of medical care used for treating your body is a basic human right!

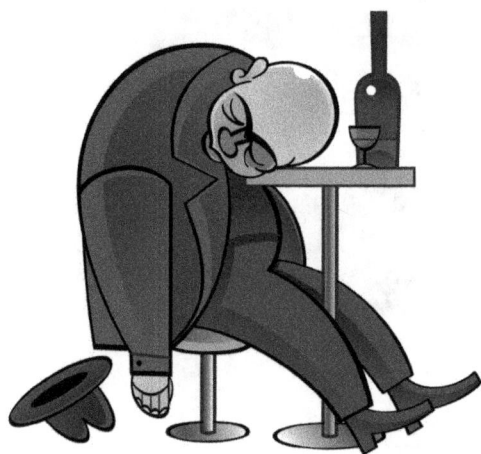

CHAPTER ONE

Alcohol

Even though the popularity of marijuana is at an all-time high and more people than are willing to admit smoke on a daily basis, you can't help but notice that there are also quite a few folks who have issues when it comes to alcohol consumption. I had always suspected that the numbers were high, but have to admit to having my mind blown by a recent scientific study on addiction that found the number of people addicted to alcohol exceeds those addicted to crack cocaine, ecstasy, methamphetamine, marijuana, oxycontin and all of the prescription drugs combined.

According to the experts while statistics on the exact number are difficult to quote with any certainty, it's conservatively estimated that there are approximately fourteen million alcohol dependent persons in the U.S. (7.4% of the population), and another seven million who have trouble controlling their consumption. Anthropologists tell us that long before drugs like crack cocaine, meth, and ecstasy, were invented alcohol earned the title and is still considered the most addictive substance known to man. If Robert O'Brien co-author of *The Encyclopedia of Alcoholism* is to be believed, there is no period in human history that is free from references to the production and consumption of intoxicating beverages.

Mr. O'Brien claims that even in pre-historic times dating back to the Neolithic period, descendants from stone-age cultures that could be described as inebriated cavemen, are known to have made fermented meads using honey as the primary ingredient for producing one of the earliest known forms of liquor. Furthermore, according to the author, since alcohol's discovery there has always been the tendency to use it in excess. It is well documented that throughout history any society where alcohol has been freely used has been affected by problems such as acute alcohol intoxication (drunkenness) and dependence. An amusing side-note that underscores this historical fact is according to some reports it was chronic alcoholism that was responsible for the death of none-other-than Attila the Hun.

Until recently social scientists were convinced that inherited genetic factors played a prominent role in causing alcohol dependence, but now they believe any person irrespective of environment, genetic background, or personality can have problems with alcohol if he/she drinks heavily for a prolonged period. Stress is an important factor. Many moderate drinkers have been known to increase their consumption of alcohol at times of bereavement, or as a response to marital, occupational, or financial stress. An interesting take on Western medicine's explanation for the underlying cause is Chinese medicine's assertion that substance abuse and addiction are a result of a mental/spiritual imbalance that the ancient medicine refers to as disturbed Shen.

According to Chinese medical theory addiction and overindulgence are merely symptoms of a deep-rooted spiritual imbalance that occurs when a person's mind and spirit are in disharmony. Traditional Chinese medicine further explains that the conflict between one's psyche and subliminal self can only be resolved when the focus of treatment goes beyond merely treating the physical complications that are inherent to the illnesses associated with the different forms of substance abuse, and focuses on restoring balance by reconnecting the mind, body, and spirit.

In order to accomplish this, traditional Chinese medicine uses herbal medicines that tranquilize the spirit and calm the Shen. In addition to treating the physical illness (patient's chief complaint), detoxifying the organs (the liver and kidneys) that filter impurities from the blood is an important part of the overall treatment. Emphasis is also placed on practicing some form of meditation either standing, sitting or moving (commonly known as Tai Chi Chuan or Chi Kung), which is also an important part of the treatment plan based on its proven ability to nurture the spirit and harmonize the emotions.

Let's Look at Some Facts about Alcohol Abuse

Among the grim statistics that clearly speak to the hazards of too much alcohol consumption is the fact that there are approximately eighty-eight-thousand deaths attributable to excessive alcohol use each year in the United States. This makes excessive alcohol use the third leading lifestyle-related cause of death for the nation. Excessive alcohol use is responsible for two and one half million years of potential life lost annually, or an average of about thirty years of potential life lost for each death. Excessive drinking notably "binge drinking," increases the risk of many harmful health conditions and alcohol related injuries such as:

- Traffic injuries, falls, drowning, burns, and unintentional firearm injuries.
- Violence, including child maltreatment, intimate, and partner violence. About thirty-five percent of victims report that offenders are under the influence of alcohol. Alcohol use is also associated with two out of three incidents of intimate partner violence. Studies have also shown that alcohol is a leading factor in child maltreatment and neglect cases, and is the most frequent substance abused among these parents.
- Risky sexual behavior such as unprotected sex, sex with multiple partners, and increased risk of sexual assault which can result in unintended pregnancy or sexually transmitted diseases.
- Miscarriage and stillbirth among pregnant women, and a combination of physical and mental birth defects among children that last throughout life.

Long term excessive alcohol use can lead to the development of chronic diseases, neurological impairments and social problems. These include but are not limited to—

- Neurological problems, including dementia, stroke and neuropathy.
- Cardiovascular problems, including myocardial infarction, cardiomyopathy, atrial fibrillation and hypertension.
- Psychiatric problems, including depression, anxiety, and suicide.
- Social problems, including unemployment, lost productivity, and family problems.
- Cancer of the mouth, throat, esophagus, liver, colon, and breast. In general, the risk of cancer increases with increasing amounts of alcohol.
- Other gastrointestinal problems, such as pancreatitis and gastritis.
- Liver diseases, including—
  - Alcoholic hepatitis.
  - Cirrhosis, which is among the fifteen leading causes of all deaths in the United States.
  - Among persons with Hepatitis C virus, worsening of liver function and interference with medications used to treat this condition.

The extensive history of human beings and their use of intoxicating spirits make it only fitting that any discussion about getting high or self-induced intoxication should begin with what many experts claim is the oldest most frequently abused addictive substance. Despite some obvious differences in their approach to treatment, Eastern and Western medicine agree that alcoholism is a condition characterized by habitual compulsive long-term consumption of alcohol, and the development of withdrawal symptoms when drinking is suddenly stopped.

There is also a shared belief between the two types of medicine that development of alcohol dependence can be divided into four distinct stages which are described in the guidelines that follow. The four stages can also be used to self-evaluate one's own alcohol consumption.

Stage One:
Tolerance increases, and the person is able to
drink more and more alcohol before
experiencing its ill effects.

Stage Two:
The drinker experiences memory lapses
relating to events that occur during
the drinking episode.

Stage Three:
There is a loss of self-control over the use of alcohol and
the drinker can no longer be certain of his/her ability to
discontinue drinking whenever he/she wants.

Stage Four:
There are prolonged binges of intoxication, and the
drinker begins to suffer observable mental
and physical complications.

Normally, there is a correlation between an alcoholic's stage of dependence and the severity of the alcohol-related diseases he/she is likely to suffer. For example, during the early stages of alcohol dependence (stage one or two), the alcoholic is more likely to experience less severe alcohol-related illnesses such as: hangover, pancreatitis, ulcers, and indigestion; however, as addiction progresses to the advanced stages of the disease (stages three and four) the alcoholic becomes more susceptible to life-threatening illnesses such as liver disease and cancer.

Slaying the Dragon provides herbal prescriptions used in traditional Chinese medicine for treating major and minor health issues associated with all of the different stages of drinking. Due to variances in symptoms from one person to another, in most cases there are several different formulas for treating a particular illness. Your selection of one formula over another should be based on which formula has the greatest number of therapeutic actions or indications that match the patient's symptoms.

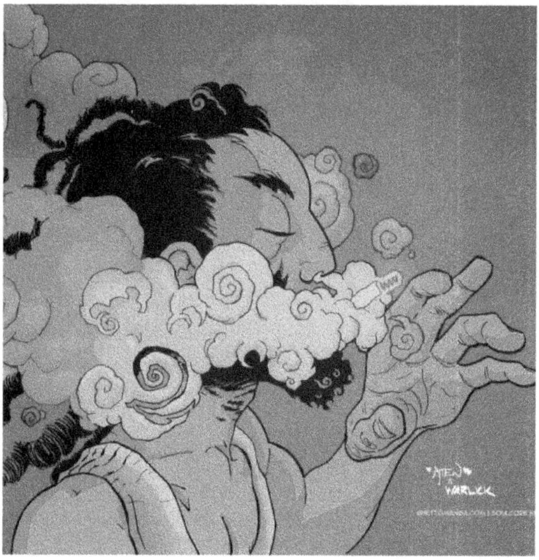

CHAPTER TWO

Drugs

In his book *An Intimate History of Humanity,* Theodore Zeldin claims it doesn't matter whether you study primordial, medieval, or modern history, regardless of the culture or civilization, there's ample evidence that human beings have been getting stoned on narcotic substances.

Long before today's modern drug culture existed even the most primitive beings are known to have used plant extracts and other botanical ingredients that were ingested, smoked, drunk, or inhaled -- either for medicinal purposes, or simply for the pleasure of getting high.

Not unlike his primordial ancestors, modern man indulges in the pleasures of euphoria for precisely the same reasons, to enhance bodily sensations and induce sensorial gratification of an aesthetic erotic nature. If they're honest most people who use drugs recreationally will admit that they enjoy using drugs because while they're under the influence of their drug of choice music sounds better, colors are brighter, and sex/orgasm is more intense.

What could be bad about something that intensifies sexual sensitivity, vamps-up music, and makes good food taste even better? Well hold on, there is a downside.

Even though this should not be considered an attempt to lecture anyone about life-style choices and the potential pit falls of substance abuse and addiction. Nevertheless, I would be remiss if I didn't remind anyone who gets high to use caution in order to avoid being devoured by what has aptly been described as the beast. If you have any doubts about the veracity of the monster you don't have to take my word for it, ask any junkie!

Let's Look at Some Facts about Drug Abuse

The importance of recognizing signs of trouble before drug use becomes problematic is what prompted me to provide the information that follows which should serve as a flashing red light. The list of symptoms is followed by a description of the effects associated with some familiar drugs. The list can be useful in several different ways:

1. When someone is seriously stoned, but there's uncertainty about which particular drug he/she has taken, matching the person's symptoms with the corresponding list of symptoms can help to determine which drug he/she may have taken.
2. When the identity of the drug that was taken is known, the list of symptoms can help to recognize the signs of serious trouble or possible overdose.

Warning Signs

Recreational drug use usually starts with casual or social use of a drug on the weekend and occasionally at parties. For some people getting high becomes a habit, and their drug use becomes more and more frequent. As time passes there may be warning signs such as needing larger doses of the drug to get high. If the situation progresses they may need the drug just to feel good. As drug use increases it becomes increasingly difficult to go without the drug. Stopping may cause intense cravings and make them feel physically ill. Other warning signs include the following:

- doing things to obtain the drug that you normally wouldn't do, such as stealing.
- driving or doing other risky activities when you're under the influence of the drug.
- failing in your attempts to stop using the drug.
- feeling that you have to use the drug regularly — this can be daily or even several times a day.
- feeling that you need the drug to deal with your problems.
- focusing more and more time and energy on getting and using the drug.
- making certain that you maintain a supply of the drug.
- spending money on the drug, even though you can't afford it.

The particular signs and symptoms of drug use and dependence vary depending on the type of drug. You might be able to tell that a family member or a friend is using or abusing a particular drug based on the physical and behavioral signs and symptoms associated with that drug. Let's review a few of the major drug types to compare signs of use.

Marijuana and hashish

Although it's possible to develop a psychological addiction to cannabis compounds, including tetrahydrocannabinol (THC) found in marijuana and hashish, people who are addicted to weed don't actually have a chemical dependence on the drug even though they may feel the need to use it on a regular basis.

Signs of use:

- A heightened sense of visual, auditory and taste perception
- Decreased coordination
- Difficulty concentrating
- Increased appetite (munchies)
- Increased blood pressure and heart rate
- Paranoid thinking
- Poor memory
- Red eyes
- Slowed reaction time

Barbiturates and benzodiazepines

Barbiturates and benzodiazepines are prescription central nervous system depressants. Pheno-barbital, amobarbital (Amytal) and secobarbital (Seconal) are examples of barbiturates. Benzo-diazepines include tranquilizers, such as diazepam (Valium), alprazolam (Xanax), lorazepam (Ativan), clonazepam (Klonopin) and chlordiazepoxide (Librium).

Signs of use:

- Confusion
- Depression
- Dizziness
- Drowsiness
- Lack of coordination
- Memory problems

- Slurred speech
- Slowed breathing and decreased blood pressure

Methamphetamines, cocaine, etc.

Stimulants are a class of drugs that include amphetamines, cocaine, methamphetamines, and methylphenidate (Ritalin).

Signs of use:

- Decreased appetite
- Depression as the drug wears off
- Euphoria
- Increased heart rate, blood pressure and temperature
- Insomnia
- Irritability
- Nasal congestion and damage to the mucous membrane of the nose in users who snort drugs
- Paranoia
- Rapid speech
- Restlessness
- Weight loss

Club drugs

Club drugs are drugs commonly used by teens and young adults at clubs, concerts and parties. Examples include Ecstasy (MDMA), GHB, Rohypnol (roofies) and ketamine. These drugs are not all classified in the same category, but they share some similar effects.

Signs of use:

- A heightened or altered sense of sight, sound and taste
- Amphetamine-like effects (with ketamine and Ecstasy)
- An exaggerated feeling of great happiness or well-being (euphoria)
- Decreased coordination
- Drowsiness and loss of consciousness (with GHB and Rohypnol)
- Increased or decreased heart rate and blood pressure
- Memory problems or loss of memory

- Poor judgment
- Reduced inhibitions

GHB and Rohypnol can be dangerous. At high doses, they can cause seizures, coma and death. The danger increases when these drugs are taken with alcohol. Because they affect consciousness and memory and they're easy to give to someone without his/her knowledge or consent, these drugs are both commonly used as date-rape drugs. One particular danger of club drugs is that the liquid, pill or powder forms of these drugs available on the street often contain unknown substances that can be harmful, including other illegally manufactured or pharmaceutical drugs.

Hallucinogens

Use of hallucinogens produces different signs and symptoms depending on the drug. The most common hallucinogens are lysergic acid diethlamide (LSD) and phencyclidine (PCP).

Signs of use:
- Confusion
- Constipation
- Depression
- Flashbacks, even years later are a re-experience of the hallucinations
- Greatly reduced perception of reality, for example, interpreting input from one of your senses as another, such as hearing colors
- Hallucinations
- High blood pressure

Narcotic painkillers

Opioids are narcotic, painkilling drugs produced naturally from opium or made synthetically. This class of drugs includes heroin, morphine, codeine, methadone and oxycodone (oxycontin).

Signs of use:
- Needle marks (if injecting drugs)
- Nodding

- Permanent mental changes in perception
- Rapid heart rate
- Reduced sense of pain
- Sedation
- Signs of narcotic use and dependence
- Slowed breathing
- Tremors

If you or someone you care about has a problem with drugs that is out of control, get help! The sooner you seek help, the greater your chances are for a long-term recovery. For those suffering from a specific drug-related disease, you may be helped by using one of the Chinese herbal formulas in this book for treating that disease.

The Chinese Plague

It's well proven that our understanding of a subject deepens when we know a little bit about its history. That said; let's take a quick look at Mao Tse Tong's Great Leap Forward and Chinese medicine's role in the Cultural Revolution. Hopefully this brief overview will provide some insight into the five-thousand-year-old medicine's role in treating addiction as well as China's no-nonsense approach in its war on drugs...

When opium was first introduced into China around the seventh century, usurious pricing and a limited supply made indulging in the pleasures of the euphoria-inducing drug beyond the means of everyone except the Emperor and the Chinese elite who more often than not were residents of the imperial court. As production increased, opium became more affordable and soon the mind-altering narcotic began spreading to all segments of Chinese society.

By the early nineteenth century under British proprietorship, the opium trade had developed into a highly lucrative, multi-national industry. The practice of using opium as a trade commodity, in exchange for tea and silk, was part of a British scheme to entice growing numbers of Chinese citizens to smoke the pernicious drug in order to create more addicts and increase China's dependence on the dreaded poppy. British poppy farms and opium processing plants, capable of producing large quantities of the drug, by no mere coincidence, were strategically located in India, which allowed for speedy delivery to the China market.

In addition to its well-known reputation for gambling and prostitution, Shanghai was also the major distribution point for opium and the city's fortunes rested on trafficking the illicit drug. As Great Britain ramped up production to satisfy the demands of an expanding Chinese market, opium was being grown, processed, and exported in plentiful supply, and it's estimated that as much as thirty to forty percent of China's population began smoking the addictive narcotic on a regular basis.

By 1839 the number of men, women, and children strung-out on the pipe had reached such epidemic proportions that irrefutable evidence of opium's addictive nature and the damage it was inflicting on millions of Chinese citizens could no longer be ignored. For China "the flower of joy" a euphemism often used to describe the addictive plant, had become a national nightmare. The ruinous effect of the drug on the Chinese population prompted government officials in the southern city of Canton to seize and destroy tons of the poisonous cargo and/order an end to its importation. China's refusal to comply with British demands for financial compensation sparked the beginning of history's most famous Sino-European conflict, commonly referred to as the Opium Wars.

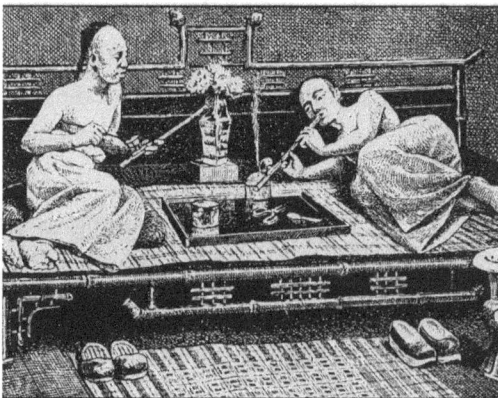

The first of the two drug wars which pitted China against Great Britain lasted from 1839-1842. Fourteen years later, a second war was fought against both Britain and France that lasted from 1856-1860. Despite a valiant effort, superior Western military forces defeated a grossly inferior Chinese army and brought China to her knees. Following the two crushing defeats at the hands of European adversaries, China would be subjected to Western domination for the better part of a century. The signing of the Treaty of Nanjing, which gave control of Hong Kong to Great Britain, was considered part of the spoils of war. The document's signing allowed England to exert even more control over Chinese affairs and tighten their financial strangle-hold on the twice-defeated Asian nation.

In the ensuing years smoking dope became so common throughout China that a lot of Westerners believed opium dens were simply an endemic feature of Chinese culture. After almost a century under foreign domination, the nation that had invented gunpowder and perfected porcelain, silk, and tea production, to become one of the wealthiest nations on earth, was reduced to a third world country, whose epidemic drug addiction was a major contributing factor to the wide-spread poverty and starvation that had created what can only be described as a national crisis.

Faced with an economy in shambles and deep-rooted moral decay that was a by-product of wide-spread drug use and government corruption; one of the first decrees of Chairman Mao Tse Tung's Revolutionary Government, following the Communist takeover in 1949, was the formation of a state-sponsored rehabilitation program in an effort to put an end to the wide-spread addiction to opium that had become rampant throughout all segments of Chinese society. As the government began tackling the daunting task of restoring sobriety to an estimated sixty to seventy million of its opium-addicted citizens—miraculously despite over-whelming odds—five years was all that was needed to virtually eliminate the drug problem that just a few years earlier had threatened to decimate a large portion of the Chinese population.

Credit for the speedy turn-around can be attributed to three things: the government's demand that all addicts enter a government-sponsored detoxification program, the use of traditional Chinese medicine as the primary method of treatment, and a requirement that recovering addicts enroll in a political re-education program that decriminalized addiction and promoted the idea that addiction is an illness, and addicts were merely victims of unscrupulous Western profiteers.

Armed with a government decree backed by military force, all opium dens were ordered closed. The closing of the iniquitous establishments was followed by the issuing of a government order that demanded the penalty of death for anyone found guilty of trafficking the illicit drug. In cases of non-compliance it was not uncommon for members of the revolutionary army to drag owners of the illegal smoking parlors from their establishments into the street, unceremoniously execute them, and leave their bloody corpses in public view as a reminder of the consequences for anyone who dared to commit a similar offense!

When we think about China's technological advances in the past fifty years, it boggles the mind when you consider that it was only a generation or so ago that the Chinese government had to resort to military force in order to prevent wide-spread opium addiction from bringing the modern day industrial giant to its knees.

From Beijing to the Big Apple

(from the opium den to the crack-house)

Fast forward to the United States a couple generations later and although preferences may have changed when it comes to the current drug of choice, the same socio-pathogenic virus that infected and almost completely devastated China has mutated, reinvented itself and is morbidly infecting all segments of today's modern high tech society.

Even though drugs like methamphetamine, heroin, crack cocaine, oxycontin and a slew of prescription medicines are the drugs of choice in today's drug culture, one can't help but notice the striking similarities.

In modern times it would be difficult to find a more poignant example of the destructive nature of pervasive drug use than New York City in the 1970's. Not only was heroin addiction and drug-related crime beyond the control of law enforcement, drugs were openly sold on practically every street corner of Manhattan's Lower East Side. When junkies weren't nodding out, they were stealing, robbing, and breaking and entering to feed their habit. Driven by their addiction, addicts were committing crimes against neighbors, friends, and loved ones that often ended in violence. In the South Bronx and Harlem the situation was at least as bad and by some estimates even worse.

In an effort to restore sanity and return to the days when people could safely walk the streets without fearing for their lives, community activists in the South Bronx began searching for a solution to try and curtail the increasing number of addicts, and reduce the drug-related crime and violence that had justifiably earned the beleaguered borough a reputation for being among the most dangerous places on earth.

After hearing reports about Mao Tse Tung's Revolutionary government's success, using traditional Chinese medicine to treat millions of its opium-addicted citizens following the communist take-over in 1949, the Young Lord's Party, a Puerto Rican nationalist group from New York's South Bronx, began exploring the possibility of using the ancient medicine to fight the epidemic heroin addiction that was destroying their once vibrant community. As the growing number of addicts continued to spread like wildfire through New York's largest Nuyorican neighborhood, there was increased pressure for the young revolutionaries to develop a drug treatment program in order to slow down the spread of the virulent disease that was mercilessly destroying lives with total disregard for age or gender. As the situation continued to spiral out of control, there was an increased sense of urgency, as frustration reached the boiling point. Acting on the adage "drastic time's call for drastic measures," the decision was made to take over the psychiatric division of Lincoln Hospital and convert the mental health unit into a much-needed drug treatment facility.

Following the takeover tensions rose to dangerous levels as the stand-off between the Young Lords and a heavily-armed New York City Police Department dragged-on for several days. Fortunately, a willingness on the part of Lincoln Hospital administrators to negotiate with the community activist group helped to avoid a situation with potentially deadly consequences.

What began as a hostile take-over was in fact, the first step in the creation of the acupuncture, drug-free detoxification program that in future years would become famous worldwide for developing the five-needle-auricular-acupuncture-protocol for treating drug addiction.

As the number of addicts successfully treated with the previously unknown Asian healing art steadily increased, positive reports about the ancient medicine spread throughout the community, and much to the dismay of crooked cops, drug dealers and pimps, there was a noticeable decrease in the demand for heroin.

Detox, which primarily involved the use of auricular acupuncture (ear points) was on an out-patient basis and normally lasted three to five days. Following withdrawal, patients were encouraged to use Chinese herbal formulas to help restore energy levels and treat the residual damage to their bodies that is often a result of long-term substance abuse. P r a c t i c i n g physical therapies like Tai Chi or Chi Kung was also highly recommended as part of recovery, to help reestablish emotional and spiritual balance. The success of the program can be attributed to the unprecedented community involvement, and the fact that the program was created and run by members of the community which empowered local citizens and made them feel they had a vested interest in its success.

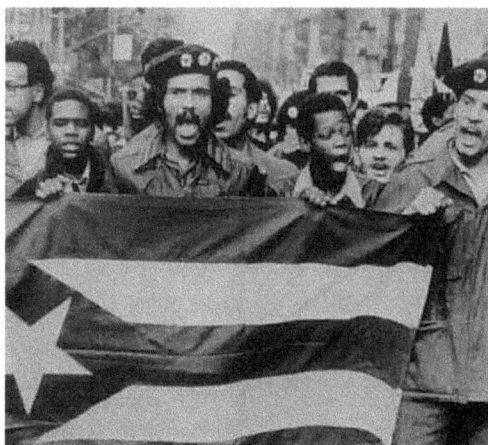

The story of the Young Lord's, the Puerto Rican revolutionary group that evolved from street gang to become a political force in the 1960's is truly amazing. Decades later the Nuyorican freedom fighters continue to garner the respect and admiration of a whole new generation of Puerto Ricans. Even though there's no question they deserve much of the credit for the creation of the now famous Lincoln Detox Program recognition for the program's success is also owed to a long list of volunteers. This list includes acupuncturists, western-trained physicians and community members, some ex-addicts and gang leaders. The common thread that joined this diverse group together was a shared belief that drug treatment facilities should be community based, and that detoxification and rehabilitation from addiction should be completely drug-free.

It is highly unlikely that the volunteers, who were instrumental in establishing the community drug treatment program, realized in future years it would serve as a model for detox programs using traditional Chinese medicine throughout the world. The Institute of Traditional Chinese Medicine New York City, of which I am an alumnus, was founded by one of the Lincoln Detox Program's original members. In the years following the programs creation in 1974, treating addiction with traditional Chinese medicine has become a topic of institutional discussion as clinics worldwide have replicated the detoxification procedures that were first developed in what has come to be known as the Lincoln Detox Program.

So that's my story—about how I became involved with Chinese medicine. As a third-generation supporter of the use of Chinese medicine (acupuncture/herbalism) in medically under-served, mostly minority communities, I support its inclusion as part of a federally-funded community-based health care system for treating all forms of illness, including alcoholism, drug abuse and addiction. As of this writing the struggle continues to establish comprehensive, affordable, drug-free rehabilitative medical treatment for people of average and low income who suffer from addiction and substance abuse.

Anyone interested in learning more about Chinese medicine and other integrative physical therapies (used for detox and rehabilitation), in drug-free traditional Chinese medical drug and alcohol treatment programs, should contact the following organizations:

- The National Acupuncture Detoxification Association, website: www.acudetox.com
- Tai Chi, Qigong (Chi Kung), and Addictions, website: http://worldtaichiday.org/life_sports_Benefits_tai_chi/ tai_chi_and_ addictions.html
- Yoga Therapy for Addiction and Alcoholism Treatment, website: http://oceanbreezerecovery.org/drug-treatment-center/ addiction-therapy/yoga/
- How Yoga Can Help During Drug and Alcohol Rehab Treatment, website: http://www.recoveryranch.com/articles/recovery-at-the-ranch/yoga-help-during-drug-and-alcohol-rehab-treatment/

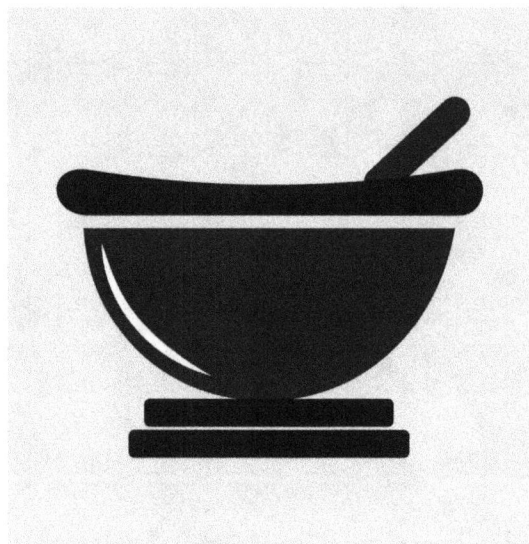

CHAPTER THREE

Chinese Herbs used to Treat Diseases/Illnesses Associated with Substance Abuse

Within this chapter you will find an alphabetical listing of the illnesses associated with alcohol and drug use as well as information on formulas that can be used to treat them. There will be a brief clinical description for each illness followed by Chinese herbal prescription(s) used for treatment. Next to each prescription I provide processing instructions that explain how the prescription is traditionally used to treat the disease, along with dosage information.

I should mention there are several illnesses discussed in this chapter that are sexually transmitted diseases (STD). If you're wondering why I've included information for treating STD it's because people who are intoxicated or stoned on drugs are more likely to engage in risky sexual behavior and unprotected sex. I feel it is important to include formulas for treating some of the most common sexually-transmitted diseases namely: candida, gonorrhea, herpes, and syphilis.

The following is an alphabetical listing with the page number of where you will find the illnesses discussed in this chapter:

Typically Chinese herbal formulas are available in raw herb form or the raw herb can be powdered by your herb supplier. The raw herb can be prepared into tea (we call that a decoction), while the powdered herb can be used to make capsules (by adding the powder to 00-sized capsules) or simply adding a heaping teaspoon of powder to four to eight ounces of smoothie or juice and drunk one to two times daily. Some formulas are available in patented pill formulas that are manufactured in China and are somewhat easier and more convenient to use; however, generally speaking, they are less potent than prescriptions prepared from raw ingredients. You can compensate for this lack of potency by taking a larger number of pills; however we encourage beginners to follow the manufacturer's recommended dosage. The drawback to taking herbs in pill form are that they are more costly than raw herbs made into tea, and typically more time is needed for the medicine to take effect while the pills are being broken down in the stomach and assimilated by the body.

Because of variances in symptoms from one person to another, in most cases I have provided several different prescriptions for treating a particular illness. Your selection of one formula over another should be based on which formula has the greatest number of therapeutic actions or indications that match the patient's symptoms.

Finally… I advise anyone who makes the decision to use Chinese herbal medicine as part of an integrative approach to conventional Western treatment or as the primary method for treating an illness, to exercise prudence and to share that information with your primary-care physician, especially if you're taking any kind of Western prescription medication.

❦

ALCOHOL POISONING

Most of us don't need to be reminded about the consequences of injecting too much of a narcotic drug like heroin into our bodies, but strangely, far too often we either fail to realize or ignore the fact that when alcohol is consumed in large amounts over a short period of time, like the drug overdose, death can be the result. It's called alcohol poisoning.

The signs and symptoms of acute alcohol poisoning, are as follows:
- When a person is known to have consumed alcohol in large quantities
- The person is cold and clammy, with pale or bluish skin
- The person's breathing is abnormally slow (ten seconds or more between each breath)
- The person vomits while passed out and does not awaken during or after

Immediate steps to preform:

- Try to wake the person by loudly calling his/her name, by slapping their face, or pinching their skin
- Check the person's breathing
- Turn the person on his/her side to prevent choking on vomit
- Do not leave the person alone
- If alcohol poisoning is suspected, call 911

Remember that in extreme cases, overindulgence of alcohol can cause a loss of consciousness and death! This is a medical emergency that requires professional medical help.

Once the person has survived the initial crisis, traditional Chinese medicine uses one particular formula to successfully treat victims of alcohol poisoning. Zhu Ru Wen Dan Tang will treat the symptoms of alcohol poisoning, such as relieving chest congestion, settling the stomach, replenishing body fluids and relieving intoxication.

Zhu Ru Wen Dan Tang
Bamboo Decoction to Warm the Gallbladder

Therapeutic Actions
Clears heat, dissolves phlegm, regulates Chi, calms the Shen (spirit), relieves chest congestion, settles the stomach, replenishes body fluid and relieves intoxication.

Preparation
Traditionally, this formula was used in the raw form to prepare a decoction; however, for those who have not developed the taste for harsh teas, we suggest the user have the ingredients ground into a fine powder by his/her herb supplier, and then store the powder in a brown or amber glass bottle with a lid. Store it in a cool environment free of sunlight and moisture until needed — do not refrigerate.

Dosage for Tang or Decoction

Drink four ounces of the warm strained decoction (tea), three times during the day as needed.

Dosage for Powder

This formula should be taken twice daily. The powder can be taken in several different ways. Make a smoothie, by adding twenty to thirty grams of the powder to eight ounces of juice smoothie, mix well, and drink. If that is an issue we recommend adding twenty to thirty grams of the powdered herbs to 00-size capsules. For more detailed instructions, follow the step-by-step guide for preparing a smoothie or capsules discussed in Chapter Five.

Herbal Ingredients

Grams	Chinese Herb	Botanical Name	Common Name
2.4	Ban Xia 半夏	*Pinellia Ternata*	Half Summer
6	Chai Hu 柴胡	*Bupleurum*	Bupleurum
2.4	Chen Pi 陳皮	*Citrus Reticulate*	Tangerine Peel
2.4	Fu Ling 茯苓	*Poria Cocos*	Tuckahoe
0.9	Gan Cao 甘草	*Glycyrrhiza Uralensis*	Licorice Root
1.5	Huang Lian 黃連	*Coptis Chinensis*	Coptis Root
6	Jie Geng 桔梗	*Platycodon*	Platycodon
15	Ren Shen 人参	*Panax Ginseng*	Ginseng
2.4	Xiang Fu 香附	*Cyperus Rotundus*	Nutgrass
6	Zhi Shi 炒枳實	*Citrus Aurantium*	Bitter Orange
6	Zhu Ru 竹茹	*Bambusa Breviflora*	Bamboo

Contraindication

This formula should not be used by pregnant women.

🍁

ANEMIA

Anemia is a condition in which the concentration of the oxygen-carrying pigment hemoglobin in the blood is below normal. The four main types are Aplastic, Iron-deficiency, Hemolytic and Megaloblastic.

1. Aplastic anemia is a result of failed formation and division of stem-cells in the bone marrow causing a drop in the number of red blood cells. Some common causes are:

    ■ treatment of cancer with radiation therapy or anti-cancer drugs

    ■ long term exposure to benzene (a constituent of gasoline) or insecticides

    ■ moderate to high doses of nuclear radiation (from radio-active fall-out or nuclear explosion)

2. Iron-deficiency anemia is a result of a lack of iron which prevents the bone marrow from making sufficient hemoglobin for the red cells. Some common causes are:

    ■ heavy menstrual bleeding

    ■ persistent internal bleeding

    ■ poor absorption as a result of surgical removal of part of or all of the stomach

    ■ a diet deficient in iron

3. Hemolytic anemia occurs when red cell production is normal, but in which there is an abnormally high rate of cell destruction. A common cause is:

    ■ usually an inherited condition

4. Megaloblastic anemia is a result of a vitamin deficiency which causes the bone marrow to produce red cells that are larger than normal and have a reduced oxygen carrying capacity. Some common causes are:

    ■ deficiency of vitamin B12 or folic acid

    ■ removal of part of the small intestine and Crohn's disease

By far the most common form of anemia worldwide is iron deficiency anemia that's a result of deficiency of iron, an essential component of hemoglobin.

The symptoms common to all of the different forms of anemia result from the reduced oxygen-carrying capacity of the blood. Their severity depends on how low the hemoglobin concentration in the blood is. Some common symptoms are bruising easily, bleeding gums, or nosebleeds. Other more severe symptoms include parlor, headache, lethargy, and shortness of breath.

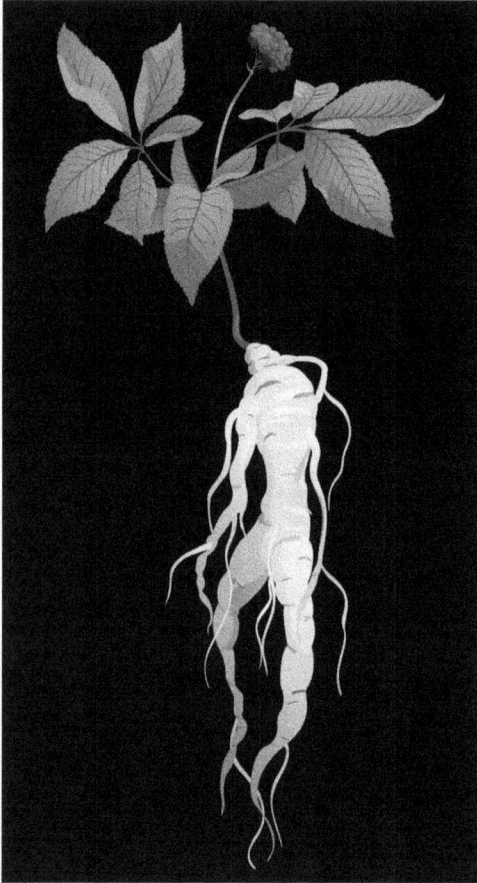

Anemia can also be a result of excessive alcohol consumption and can occur as a side effect of cirrhosis when blood flow becomes slowed in the portal vein. This can cause blood to back-up in the gastro-intestinal tract, which in turn creates hemorrhoids, esophageal varices, and intestinal lesions.

In traditional Chinese medicine anemia is referred to as "deficient blood." A prescription that has proven effectiveness in treating this underlying deficiency is the four ingredient classical formula known as Si Wu Tang. The joining of forces of the "four gentlemen" a euphemism, often used to describe the herbal quartet, is a standard treatment method for a host of blood disorders, including anemia. The four mutually assisting ingredients that make-up the ancient prescription nourish and enrich the blood, improve circulation, and regulate its viscosity.

The following herbal prescriptions can be used to treat anemia; also included are processing instructions and the formula's therapeutic action.

RAW HERB FORMULAS
Si Wu Tang
Four-Substance Decoction

Therapeutic Actions
This formula is used to treat the symptoms of anemia, including postpartum anemia, and irregular menstruation. In TCM this formula is famous for its ability to nourish the blood and regulate blood circulation. While it treats all forms of anemia, it is particularly effective treating iron deficiency anemia as well as megaloblastic anemia. For best results, when treating megaloblastic anemia you may want to consider taking vitamin B12 and folic acid supplements.

Preparation
Traditionally, this formula was used in the raw form to prepare a decoction; however, for those who have not developed the taste for harsh teas, we suggest the user have the ingredients ground into a fine powder by his/her herb supplier, and then store the powder in a brown or amber glass bottle with a lid. Store it in a cool environment free of sunlight and moisture until needed — do not refrigerate.

*Dosage Note
The gram weight to be used in this formula is listed with a minimum/maximum range. This prescription should be prepared by using the lower dosage and only increase dosage to achieve stronger results when needed.

Dosage for Tang or Decoction

Drink four ounces of the warm strained decoction (tea), three times during the day as needed.

Dosage for Powder

This formula should be taken twice daily. The powder can be taken in several different ways. Make a smoothie, by adding twenty to thirty grams of the powder to eight ounces of juice smoothie, mix well, and drink. If that is an issue we recommend adding twenty to thirty grams of the powdered herbs to 00-size capsules. For more detailed instructions, follow the step-by-step guide for preparing a smoothie or capsules discussed in Chapter Five.

Herbal Ingredients

Grams	Chinese Herb	Botanical Name	Common Name
9–12*	Bai Shao 白芍	*Paeonia Lactiflora*	White Peony
6–9*	Chuan Xiong 川芎	*Ligusticum*	Cnidium
9–12*	Dang Gui 當歸	*Angelica*	Angelica
12	Shu Di Huang 熟地黃	*Rehmanniae Preparata*	Rehmannia Cooked

Sheng Yu Tang

Sage-like Healing Decoction

Therapeutic Actions

This formula is used to treat the symptoms of aplastic anemia, including Chi and blood deficiency, excessive menstrual bleeding, lethargy, and weakness in the limbs. In TCM this formula is famous for its ability to nourish the blood and regulate blood circulation. While it treats all forms of anemia, it is particularly effective treating aplastic anemia.

Preparation

Traditionally, this formula was used in the raw form to prepare a decoction; however, for those who have not developed the taste for harsh teas, we suggest the user have the ingredients ground into a fine powder by his/her herb supplier, and then store the powder in a brown or amber glass bottle with a lid. Store it in a cool environment free of sunlight and moisture until needed — do not refrigerate.

Dosage for Tang or Decoction

Drink four ounces of the warm strained decoction (tea), three times during the day as needed.

Dosage for Powder

This formula should be taken twice daily. The powder can be taken in several different ways. Make a smoothie, by adding twenty to thirty grams of the powder to eight ounces of juice smoothie, mix well, and drink. If that is an issue we recommend adding twenty to thirty grams of the powdered herbs to 00-size capsules. For more detailed instructions, follow the step-by-step guide for preparing a smoothie or capsules discussed in Chapter Five.

Herbal Ingredients

Grams	Chinese Herb	Botanical Name	Common Name
15	Dang Gui 當歸	*Angelica*	Angelica
15	Huang Qin 黃芩	*Schutellaria*	Skullcap
23	Ren Shen 人参	*Panax Ginseng*	Ginseng
23	Shu Di Huang 熟地黃	*Rehmanniae Preparata*	Rehmannia Cooked

Shi Quan Da Bu Tang

All-inclusive Great Tonifying Decoction

Therapeutic Actions

This formula is used to treat the symptoms of anemia, including hemolytic anemia with lethargy. In TCM this formula is famous for its ability to nourish the blood and regulate blood circulation. While it treats all forms of anemia, it is particularly effective for treating hemolytic anemia.

Preparation

Traditionally, this formula was used in the raw form to prepare a decoction; however, for those who have not developed the taste for harsh teas, we suggest the user have the ingredients ground into a fine powder by his/her herb supplier, and then store the powder in a brown or amber glass bottle with a lid. Store it in a cool environment free of sunlight and moisture until needed — do not refrigerate.

Dosage for Tang or Decoction

Drink four ounces of the warm strained decoction (tea), three times during the day as needed.

Dosage for Powder

This formula should be taken twice daily. The powder can be taken in several different ways. Make a smoothie, by adding twenty to thirty grams of the powder to eight ounces of juice smoothie, mix well, and drink. If that is an issue we recommend adding twenty to thirty grams of the powdered herbs to 00-size capsules. For more detailed instructions, follow the step-by-step guide for preparing a smoothie or capsules discussed in Chapter Five.

Herbal Ingredients

Grams	Chinese Herb	Botanical Name	Common Name
8	Bai Shao 白芍	*Paeonia Lactiflora*	White Peony
10	Bai Zhu 白朮	*Atractylodes*	Atractylodes
5	Chuan Xiong 川芎	*Ligusticum*	Cnidium
10	Dang Gui 當歸	*Angelica*	Angelica
8	Fu Ling 茯苓	*Poria Cocos*	Tuckahoe
15	Huang Qi 黃芪	*Astragalus*	Milkvetch
8	Ren Shen 人參	*Panax Ginseng*	Ginseng
8	Rou Gui 肉桂	*Cinnamomum*	Cinnamon Bark
15	Shu Di Huang 熟地黃	*Rehmanniae Preparata*	Rehmannia Cooked
5	Zhi Gan Cao 甘草	*Glycyrrhizae*	Licorice

BACTERIAL ENDOCARDITIS

The various types of endocarditis include acute bacterial, sub-acute bacterial, fungal, and nonbacterial. In both types of bacterial endocarditis, causative microorganisms enter the bloodstream and infect the lining of the heart and valves, eventually causing damage.

Intravenous drug users are particularly susceptible to bacterial endocarditis because of the possibility of introducing bacteria and fungi from dirty syringes, and because of the risk of transmitting infection from unclean skin at the site of injection. There is a higher risk of fungal endocarditis occurring in people who have suppressed immune systems and low resistance to infection, such as sufferers of HIV.

Symptoms include fatigue, weakness, feverishness, night sweats and vague aches and pains. The patient may also suffer from severe chills, high fever, shortness of breath, and rapid or irregular heartbeat.

Diagnosis includes a blood test that is examined for bacteria and fungi as well as heart tests such as echo-cardiography and angiography. Once the diagnosis is confirmed, treatment normally consists of administering high doses of antibiotics. Treatment can last for as long as six to eight weeks.

Successful Chinese medical treatment will focus on the symptoms of bacterial endocarditis including: fatigue, weakness, night sweats, vague aches and pains, severe chills, high fever, shortness of breath, and rapid or irregular heartbeat.

The following herbal prescription can be used to treat bacterial endocarditis; also included are processing instructions and the formula's therapeutic action.

Zhi Gan Cao Tang

Honey Licorice Decoction

Therapeutic Actions

This formula is used to treat the symptoms of bacterial endocarditis, including fatigue, weakness, feverishness, night sweats, vague aches and pains, severe chills, high fever, shortness of breath, and rapid or irregular heartbeat.

Preparation

Traditionally, this formula was used in the raw form to prepare a decoction; however, for those who have not developed the taste for harsh teas, we suggest the user have the ingredients ground into a fine powder by his/her herb supplier, and then store the powder in a brown or amber glass bottle with a lid. Store it in a cool environment free of sunlight and moisture until needed — do not refrigerate.

*Preparation Notes

The herb Sheng Jiang or fresh ginger should not be cooked for longer than five minutes. Do not add it to the herbs being cooked until the last five minutes of preparation time. E Jiao should not be cooked with the rest of this formula. After finishing the cooking process, add in the E Jiao, stir well to dissolve, and then steep the decoction for fifteen minutes, and strain off the herbs.

Dosage for Tang or Decoction

Drink four ounces of the warm strained decoction (tea), three times during the day as needed.

Dosage for Powder

This formula should be taken twice daily. The powder can be taken in several different ways. Make a smoothie, by adding twenty to thirty grams of the powder to eight ounces of juice smoothie, mix well, and drink. If that is an issue we recommend adding twenty to thirty grams of the powdered herbs to 00-size capsules. For more detailed instructions, follow the step-by-step guide for preparing a smoothie or capsules discussed in Chapter Five.

Herbal Ingredients

Grams	Chinese Herb	Botanical Name	Common Name
6-10 pieces	Da Zao 大 棗	*Ziziphus Jujuba*	Jujube
6	E Jiao* 阿胶	*Equus Asinus*	Ass-Hide Glue
9	Gui Zhi 桂枝	*Cinnamomum*	Cinnamon
9	Huo Ma Ren 火麻仁	*Fructus Cannabis*	Hemp Seeds
9	Mai Men Dong 麦冬	*Ophiopogon*	Winter Wheat
6	Ren Shen 人参	*Panax Ginseng*	Ginseng
9	Sheng Jiang* 生姜	*Zingiber*	Ginger Sliced
30	Shu Di Huang 熟地黃	*Rehmanniae Preparata*	Rehmannia Cooked
12	Zhi Gan Cao 甘草	*Glycyrrhizae*	Licorice

🍁

CANDIDIASIS

Candidiasis is an infection by the fungus candida albicans, inside of the vagina or less commonly, on other areas of mucus membrane such as inside of the mouth or on moist skin. The infection is also known as thrush or moniliasis.

Vaginal candidiasis may cause a thick white cottage-cheese-like discharge from the vagina and/or irritation in the area, which may cause discomfort when passing urine. If the fungus is present within the mouth, it produces sore creamy-yellow, raised patches. It can also spread to other moist areas of the body, such as the skin folds in the groin or under the breasts in women.

Candida infection of the penis which is more common among uncircumcised than circumcised males, is usually the result of sexual intercourse with an infected partner. Infection of the penis usually results in balanitis (infection of the head of the penis).

Chinese herbal prescriptions that contain anti-fungal herbs will usually clear up the problem, but the infection may reoccur as a result of reinfection by a sexual partner. Therefore, the treatment of any and all partners is highly recommended.

Successful Chinese medical treatment of candidiasis depends on the use of herbal formulas that contain potent anti-fungal herbs that will treat the infection, relieve irritation of the vaginal area or mouth, and dry up sores or raised patches.

The following prescriptions can be used to treat candidiasis. For each prescription, I will provide processing instructions and the formulas therapeutic action.

RAW HERB FORMULA
Liang Ge San
Cool the Diaphragm Powder

Therapeutic Actions
This formula is used to clear up the infection candida albicans; it treats many types of infection including candidiasis, herpes labiales, and meningitis.

Preparation
Traditionally, this formula was used in the raw form to prepare a decoction; however, for those who have not developed the taste for harsh teas, we suggest the user have the ingredients ground into a fine powder by his/her herb supplier, and then store the powder in a brown or amber glass bottle with a lid. Store it in a cool environment free of sunlight and moisture until needed — do not refrigerate.

*Preparation Note
The Bo He should not be cooked with the rest of this formula. After finishing the cooking process, add in the Bo He, stir well, and then steep the decoction for fifteen minutes, and then strain off the herbs.

Dosage for Tang or Decoction
Drink four ounces of the warm strained decoction (tea), once or twice during the day as needed.

Dosage for Powder

This formula should be taken once or twice daily. The powder can be used in several different ways. Make a smoothie, by adding twenty to thirty grams of the powder to eight ounces of juice smoothie, mix well, and drink. If that is an issue we recommend adding twenty to thirty grams of the powdered herbs to 00-size capsules. For more detailed instructions, follow the step-by-step guide for preparing a smoothie or capsules discussed in Chapter Five.

Herbal Ingredients

Grams	Chinese Herb	Botanical Name	Common Name
5	Bo He* 薄荷	*Mentha Haplocalyx*	Mint
9	Da Huang 大黃	*Rheum Palmatum*	Rhubarb
9	Gan Cao 甘草	*Glycyrrhiza*	Licorice
5	Huang Qin 黄芩	*Schutellaria*	Baikal Skullcap
18	Lian Qiao 连翘	*Forsythia Suspensa*	Forsythia
9	Po Xiao 芒硝	*Sal Glauberis*	Sodium Sulfate
5	Zhi Zi 栀子	*Gardenia*	Gardenia

Contraindication

Use when pregnant is contraindicated.

Note

As with all STD it is advisable to treat all sexual partners to avoid reinfection.

PATENT HERB FORMULAS

Bi Xie Sheng Shi Wan

Subdue the Dampness Teapills

Therapeutic Actions

This patent formula is used to treat infections such as candida albicans; including eczema, urticarial, poison ivy, itching, open sores, and candidiasis.

Cautions

Generally well-tolerated formula; however, long-term use can weaken the digestive system. Do not use if pregnant.

Packaged

In bottle of two hundred pills.

Dosage

Take eight pills three times daily.

Yu Dai Wan

Heal Vaginal Discharge Pill

Therapeutic Actions

This patent formula is used to treat infections such as candida albicans; including leukorrhea, vaginal discharge, trichomoniasis, and candidiasis.

Packaged

In bottle of one hundred pills.

Dosage

Take eight pills three times daily.

Note

As with all STD it is advisable to treat all sexual partners to avoid reinfection.

🍁

CIRRHOSIS

After liver cancer, cirrhosis is perhaps the most serious alcohol-related liver disease. Cirrhosis occurs when there is cell damage caused by built-up scar tissue. Because these nodules are inadequately supplied with blood, liver function is impaired, undermining its ability to effectively remove toxic substances from the blood. This distortion and scarring will lead to portal hypertension (high blood pressure in the veins from the intestines and spleen to the liver).

Approximately thirty thousand people die each year in the U.S. as a direct result of chronic liver disease and cirrhosis. Heavy alcohol consumption is the most common cause. The risk of contracting liver disease relates to the amount of alcohol consumed rather than the type, and statistically, women are more susceptible than men.

There are four main complications associated with cirrhosis, and any one of the four may signal the onset of the condition:

1. ascites which is the accumulation of fluid in the abdominal cavity (the alcoholic pot–belly), caused by low protein levels in the blood and high blood pressure in the veins leading to the liver

2. esophageal varices or enlarged veins in the wall of the esophagus, which can rupture causing vomiting of blood

3. coma resulting from the accumulation of toxic materials poisonous to the brain that are normally processed and detoxified by a healthy liver

4. and hepatoma, which is a primary cancer of liver cells, complicating chronic hepatitis with cirrhosis.

Although liver function tests may present symptoms associated with cirrhosis, diagnosis is usually confirmed by liver biopsy. Cirrhosis, which is treatable, involves slowing down cell damage by treating the complications previously mentioned, and abstaining from alcohol which can lead to substantial improvement. However, in severe cases, a liver transplant may offer the only chance of long-term cures.

Successful Chinese medical treatment depends on the use of herbal formulas that resolve the jaundice (yellowish color of the skin and eyes), reduce edema (the swelling caused by water retention), relieve mental confusion, stop hematemesis (vomiting of blood), and reduce male breast enlargement and loss of body hair. Chinese herbal medicine can effectively treat these symptoms; however, the user must refrain from the use of alcohol in order for recovery to be possible and prevent further liver damage.

All of the herbal prescriptions that follow can be used to treat cirrhosis. For each prescription, I will provide processing instructions and the formulas therapeutic action.

RAW HERB FORMULAS
Bie Jia Jian Wan
Soft-Shelled Turtle Shell Pill

Therapeutic Actions

This prescription is used to treat liver cirrhosis and liver cancer; it increases circulation of blood and Chi, relieves the body of dampness and dissolves phlegm, it softens hard masses, reduces distention and abdominal pain, and stops muscle wasting while improving the appetite.

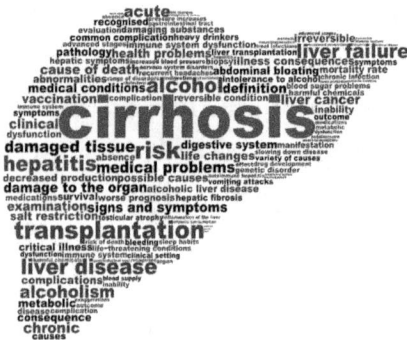

Preparation

Traditionally, this formula is used in the raw form to prepare pills or capsules; the user should have the ingredients ground into a fine powder by his/her herb supplier, and then store the powder in a brown or amber glass bottle with a lid. Store it in a cool environment free of sunlight and moisture until needed — do not refrigerate.

Dosage

This formula should be taken three times daily. The powder can be used in several different ways. Make a smoothie, by adding twenty to thirty grams of the powder to eight ounces of juice smoothie, mix well, and drink. If that is an issue we recommend adding twenty to thirty grams of the powdered herbs to 00-size capsules. For more detailed instructions, follow the step-by-step guide for preparing a smoothie or pills or capsules discussed in Chapter Five.

Herbal Ingredients

Grams	Chinese Herb	Botanical Name	Common Name
37	Bai Shao 白芍	*Paeonia Lactiflora*	White Peony
7.5	Ban Xia 半夏	*Pinellia Ternata*	Half Summer
90	Bie Jia 鳖甲	*Trionyx Sinensis*	Turtle Shell
45	Chai Hu 柴胡	*Bupleurum*	Bupleurum
22.5	Da Huang 大黄	*Rheum Palmatum*	Rhubarb
22.5	E Jiao 阿胶	*Equus Asinus*	Ass-Hide Glue
30	Lu Feng Fang 露蜂	*Nidus Vespae*	Hornet's Nest
22.5	Gan Jiang 乾薑	*Zingiber Officinale*	Ginger Dried
22.5	Gui Zhi 桂枝	*Cinnamomum*	Cinnamon
22.5	Hou Po 厚朴	*Magnolia Officinalis*	Magnolia Bark
22.5	Huang Qin 黄芩	*Schutellaria*	Skullcap
22.5	Ling Xiao Hua 凌霄花	*Flos Campsis*	Trumpet Creeper
90	Mang Xiao 芒硝	*Natrii Sulfas*	Sodium Sulfate
37	Mu Dan Pi 牡丹皮	*Paeonia Suffruticosa*	Tree Peony
45	Qiang Lang 蜣螂	*Catharsium*	Dung Beetle
22.5	Qu Mai 瞿麦	*Dianthus Superbus*	Dianthus
7.5	Ren Shen 人参	*Panax Ginseng*	Ginseng
22.5	She Gan 射干	*Belamcanda*	Blackberry Lily
22.5	Shi Wei 石韦	*Pyrosia Sheareri*	Japanese Fern
22.5	Shu Fu Chong 鼠妇虫	*Armadillidium*	Pillbug
15	Tao Ren 桃仁	*Prunus Persica*	Peach Seed
7.5	Ting Li Zi 葶苈子	*Descurainia Sophia*	Lepidum
37	Tu Bei Chong 土鳖虫	*Eupolyphaga*	Eupolyphaga

Shao Fu Zhu Yu Tang

Drive out Blood Stasis in the Lower Abdomen

Therapeutic Actions

Used for treating cirrhosis of the liver with edema (swelling of the feet and/or ankles due to water retention), lower abdominal pain, and distention (swollen abdomen).

Preparation

Traditionally, this formula was used in the raw form to prepare a decoction; however, for those who have not developed the taste for harsh teas, we suggest the user have the ingredients ground into a fine powder by his/her herb supplier, and then store the powder in a brown or amber glass bottle with a lid. Store it in a cool environment free of sunlight and moisture until needed — do not refrigerate.

Dosage for Tang or Decoction

Drink four ounces of the warm strained decoction (tea), three times during the day as needed.

Dosage for Powder

This formula should be taken twice daily. The powder can be used in several different ways. Make a smoothie, by adding twenty to thirty grams of the powder to eight ounces of juice smoothie, mix well, and drink. If that is an issue we recommend adding twenty to thirty grams of the powdered herbs to 00-size capsules. For more detailed instructions, follow the step-by-step guide for preparing a smoothie or capsules discussed in Chapter Five.

Contraindication

This formula should not be used by pregnant women.

Herbal Ingredients

Grams	Chinese Herb	Botanical Name	Common Name
6	Chi Shao 赤芍	*Paeonia Veitchii*	Red Peony
3	Chuan Xiong 川芎	*Ligusticum*	Cnidium
9	Dang Gui 當歸	*Angelica*	Angelica
0.6	Gan Jiang Chao	*Zingiberis Officinale*	Ginger Dried
	干姜	*Preparata*	Cooked
3	Hong Hua 紅花	*Carthamus*	Carthamus
3	Mo Yao 没药	*Myrrha*	Myrrh
9	Pu Huang 蒲黄炭	*Typha Angustifolia*	Bulrush
3	Rou Gui 肉桂	*Cinnamomum*	Cinnamon Bark
9	Sheng Di Huang 生地黃	*Rehmannia*	Rehmannia Dried
6	Si Gua Luo 丝瓜络	*Luffa Cylindrical*	Luffa Fiber
6	Tao Ren 桃仁	*Prunus Persica*	Peach Seed
6	Wu Ling Zhi Chao	*Trogopterius Xanthipes*	Pteropus Feces
	五灵脂	*Preparata*	Cooked
3	Wu Yao 烏藥	*Lindera Strychnifolia*	Lindera
6	Xiang Fu 香附	*Cyperus Rotundus*	Nutgrass e
1.5	Xiao Hui Xiang Chao	*Foeniculum Vulgare*	Fennel Seed
	小茴香	*Preparata*	Cooked
3	Yan Hu Suo 延胡索	*Corydalis*	Corydalis

Shu Gan Li Pi Tang

Spread the Liver and Regulate the Spleen Decoction

Therapeutic Actions

This formula treats cirrhosis, and benefits the liver, regulates the spleen, and nourishes and invigorates the blood. It reduces pain and the sensation of fullness in the chest/abdomen, also benefits insomnia, fatigue, and reduced appetite, as well as diarrhea.

Preparation

Traditionally, this formula was used in the raw form to prepare a decoction; however, for those who have not developed the taste for harsh teas, we suggest the user have the ingredients ground into a fine powder by his/ her herb supplier, and then store the powder in a brown or amber glass bottle with a lid. Store it in a cool environment free of sunlight and moisture until needed — do not refrigerate.

Dosage for Tang or Decoction

Drink four ounces of the warm strained decoction (tea), three times during the day as needed.

Dosage for Powder

This formula should be taken twice daily. The powder can be used in several different ways. Make a smoothie, by adding twenty to thirty grams of the powder to eight ounces of juice smoothie, mix well, and drink. If that is an issue we recommend adding twenty to thirty grams of the powdered herbs to 00-size capsules. For more detailed instructions, follow the step-by-step guide for preparing a smoothie or capsules discussed in Chapter Five.

Herbal Ingredients

Grams	Chinese Herb	Botanical Name	Common Name
12	Bai Zhu 白朮	*Atractylodes*	Atractylodes
12	Chai Hu 柴胡	*Bupleurum*	Bupleurum
12	Dan Shen 丹參	*Salvia Miltiorrhiza*	Salvia Root
15	Dang Shen 党參	*Codonoposis*	Codonopsis
12	He Shou Wu 何首乌	*Polygonum*	Polygonum
3	San Qi, sliced 三七	*Panax Notoginseng*	Pseudoginseng
9	Xiang Fu 香附	*Cyperus Rotundus*	Nutgrass
9	Ze Xie 澤瀉	*Alisma Orientalis*	Water Plantain

Yi Guan Jian
Linking Decoction

Therapeutic Actions
This formula can be used during the early stages of cirrhosis; it is useful when there is chest pain, abdominal distention (bloated stomach), dry mouth, acid regurgitation, and loss of weight.

Preparation
Traditionally, this formula was used in the raw form to prepare a decoction; however, for those who have not developed the taste for harsh teas, we suggest the user have the ingredients ground into a fine powder by his/her herb supplier, and then store the powder in a brown or amber glass bottle with a lid. Store it in a cool environment free of sunlight and moisture until needed — do not refrigerate.

*Dosage Note
The gram weight to be used in this formula is listed with a minimum/maximum range. This prescription should be prepared by using the lower dosage and only increase dosage to achieve stronger results when needed.

Dosage for Tang or Decoction
Drink four ounces of the warm strained decoction (tea), three times during the day as needed.

Dosage for Powder
This formula should be taken twice daily. The powder can be used in several different ways. Make a smoothie, by adding twenty to thirty grams of the powder to eight ounces of juice smoothie, mix well, and drink. If that is an issue we recommend adding twenty to thirty grams of the powdered herbs to 00-size capsules. For more detailed instructions, follow the step-by-step guide for preparing a smoothie or capsules discussed in Chapter Five.

Herbal Ingredients

Grams	Chinese Herb	Botanical Name	Common Name
9	Bei Sha Shen 北沙蔘	*Glehniae*	Glehnia
4.5	Chuan Lian Zi 川楝子	*Melia Toosendan*	Chinaberry Fruit
9	Dang Gui 當歸	*Angelica*	Angelica
9-18*	Gou Qi Zi 枸杞子	*Lycii Fructus*	Wolfberry
9	Mai Men Dong 麦冬	*Ophiopogon*	Winter Wheat
18-45*	Sheng Di Huang 生地黃	*Rehmannia*	Rehmannia Dried

Zhou Che Wan

Vessel and Vehicle Pill

Therapeutic Actions

Used for treating cirrhosis, with or without edema (swelling or puffiness due to water retention), and ascites (fluid in the chest cavity) that have caused a stoppage of either urination or bowel movement. Discontinue use of this formula once urination and bowel movement have been restored.

Preparation

Grind the ingredients into a fine powder, and store the powder in a brown or amber glass bottle with a lid. Store it in a cool environment free of sunlight and moisture until needed — do not refrigerate.

  This formula should not be taken on an empty stomach. There are several different ways that the powder can be used. A dose of the powder can be added to juice or a smoothie to drink. If that is an issue we recommend putting the powdered herbs into 00-size capsules. For more detailed instructions, follow the step-by-step guide for preparing a smoothie, pills or capsules discussed in Chapter Five.

Dosage

Add three to six grams of powder to capsules, or to eight ounces of juice or smoothie to drink once daily in the morning.

Contraindications

This formula should not be used by pregnant women. This formula is for short–term use only; prolonged use of this formula is contraindicated. This formula should not be taken on an empty stomach.

Herbal Ingredients

Grams	Chinese Herb	Botanical Name	Common Name
15	Bing Lang 槟榔	*Araca Catechu*	Betel Nut
15	Chen Pi 陳皮	*Citrus Reticulate*	Tangerine Peel
60	Da Huang 大黃	*Rheum Palmatum*	Rhubarb Root
30	Da Ji 大薊	*Euphorbia Pekinensis*	Knoxia
30	Gan Sui 甘遂	*Euphorbia Kansui*	Gansui Root
15	Mu Xiang 木香	*Aucklandiae Lappa*	Costus Root
120	Qian Niu Zi 牵牛子	*Pharbitis Nil*	Pharbitis Seed
3	Qing Fen 轻粉	*Calomelas*	Calomel
15	Qing Pi 青皮	*Citrus Reticulata Blanco*	Green Tangerine Peel
30	Yuan Hua 芫花	*Daphne Genkwa*	Lilac Daphne

PATENT HERB FORMULAS
Bu Zhong Yi Qi Tang
Central Chi Pills, Tonify Center, Increase Chi Pills

Therapeutic Actions

This patent formula is used to treat chronic diarrhea associated with cirrhosis and hepatitis; it relieves poor digestion with loose stools, chronic diarrhea, and flatulence.

Packaged

In bottle of two hundred pills.

Dosage

Take eight pills, three times per day. Dosage can be increase to twelve pills, if needed.

Fang Ji Huang Qi Wan

Stephania, Astragalus Pills

Therapeutic Actions
This patent formula is used to treat ascites due to liver cirrhosis; relieves edema and diarrhea.

Packaged
In bottle of two hundred pills.

Dosage
Take eight pills three times daily.

🍁

DELIRIUM TREMENS

People who suffer from what is commonly referred to as DTs or the shakes are usually chronic alcoholics who attempt to stop drinking and are going through withdrawal, or they're active alcoholics who need a drink and are experiencing a severe physical reaction to their bodies' craving for alcohol.

In the early stages, symptoms such as restlessness, agitation, and sleeplessness are common. Delirium tremens are also known to cause rapid heartbeat, fever, dilation of the pupils, and profuse sweating that can lead to dehydration.

The most notable symptoms are the familiar shakes or tremors, confusion, auditory and visual hallucinations where the sufferer imagines seeing and hearing things. Convulsions may also occur, and in most cases the patient appears terrified. Normally after two-three days of rest rehydration and sedation, the symptoms subside.

Although it is fairly uncommon, delirium tremens can be fatal. Therefore, before attempting alcohol withdrawal you may want to consider seeking professional medical assistance.

Successful treatment using Chinese herbal medicine depends on the use of herbal formulas that relieves restlessness, the shakes, agitation fever, profuse sweating, and enables the heart to retain a normal heartbeat The next four herbal prescriptions are all single-herb formulas that are used to effectively treat delirium tremens. The first two are Chinese Herbs. The last two, are Western herbs that were included because of the excellent ratings they receive for their effectiveness in reducing the shakes. For each prescription, I will provide its unique processing instructions and therapeutic action.

RAW HERB FORMULAS
Ge Gen Decoction
Kudzu Root Tea

Therapeutic Actions
This single-herb formula can be used to treat the symptoms of the DTs; it is primarily used to reduce tremors and the craving for alcohol.

Preparation
Traditionally, this formula was used in the raw form to prepare a decoction; however, for those who have not developed the taste for harsh teas, we suggest the user have the ingredients ground into a fine powder by his/her herb supplier, and then store the powder in a brown or amber glass bottle with a lid. Store it in a cool environment free of sunlight and moisture until needed — do not refrigerate.

Dosage for Tang or Decoction
Drink eight to twelve ounces of the warm strained decoction (tea), three times during the day as needed.

Dosage for Powder
This formula should be taken twice daily. The powder can be used in several different ways. Make a smoothie, by adding twenty to thirty grams of the

powder to eight ounces of juice smoothie, mix well, and drink. If that is an issue we recommend adding twenty to thirty grams of the powdered herbs to 00-size capsules. For more detailed instructions, follow the step-by-step guide for preparing a smoothie or capsules discussed in Chapter Five.

Herbal Ingredient

Grams	Chinese Herb	Botanical Name	Common Name
20	Ge Gen 葛根	*Radix Puerariae*	Kudzu

Shi Chang Pu Decoction
Acorus Gramineu Tea

Therapeutic Actions
This single-herb formula can be used to treat the symptoms of the DTs; it is primarily used to stop convulsions and seizures, to slow down the heart rate during treatment, and reduce the craving for alcohol.

Preparation
Traditionally, this formula was used in the raw form to prepare a decoction; however, for those who have not developed the taste for harsh teas, we suggest the user have the ingredients ground into a fine powder by his/her herb supplier, and then store the powder in a brown or amber glass bottle with a lid. Store it in a cool environment free of sunlight and moisture until needed — do not refrigerate.

Dosage for Tang or Decoction
Drink eight ounces of the warm strained decoction (tea), once during the day as needed.

Dosage for Powder
This formula should be taken twice daily. The powder can be used in several different ways. Make a smoothie, by adding twenty to thirty grams of the powder to eight ounces of juice smoothie, mix well, and drink. If that is an

issue we recommend adding twenty to thirty grams of the powdered herbs to 00-size capsules. For more detailed instructions, follow the step-by-step guide for preparing a smoothie or capsules discussed in Chapter Five.

Herbal Ingredient

Grams	Chinese Herb	Botanical Name	Common Name
10	Shi Chang Pu 石菖蒲	*Acori*	Acorus

La Jiao Tea

Cayenne Red Pepper Decoction

Therapeutic Actions

This single-herb formula can be used to treat the symptoms of the DTs, primarily used to relieve the shakes, the chills, and the crawly-sensation felt all over the body that is commonly experienced during withdrawal.

Preparation

Traditionally, this formula was used in the raw form to prepare a decoction; however, for those who have not developed the taste for harsh teas, we suggest the user have the ingredients ground into a fine powder by his/her herb supplier, and then store the powder in a brown or amber glass bottle with a lid. Store it in a cool environment free of sunlight and moisture until needed — do not refrigerate.

Dosage for Tang or Decoction

To make a cup of tea use fifteen-thirty grams of herb to eight ounces of boiling water, steep and drink the warm strained decoction (tea), once during the day or as needed.

Dosage for Powder

This formula should be taken once daily. The powder can be used in several different ways. Make a smoothie, by adding fifteen-thirty grams of the powder to eight ounces of juice smoothie, mix well, and drink. If that is an issue we recommend adding fifteen–thirty grams of the powdered herbs to 00-size capsules. For more detailed instructions, follow the step-by-step guide for preparing a smoothie or capsules discussed in Chapter Five.

*Dosage Note

The gram weight to be used in this formula is listed with a minimum/maximum range. This prescription should be prepared by using the lower dosage and only increase dosage to achieve stronger results when needed.

Herbal Ingredient

Grams	Chinese Herb	Botanical Name	Common Name
15-30*	La Jiao 辣椒	*Capsicum Annuum*	Cayenne Red Pepper

Xi Fan Lian Tea

Passion Flower Decoction

Therapeutic Actions

This single-herb formula can be used to treat the symptoms of the DTs, primarily used to relieve the tremors, spasms, shakes, insomnia, and sleep disturbances that are commonly experienced during withdrawal.

Preparation

Traditionally, this formula was used in the raw form to prepare a decoction; however, for those who have not developed the taste for harsh teas, we suggest the user have the ingredients ground into a fine powder by his/her herb supplier, and then store the powder in a brown or amber glass bottle with a lid. Store it in a cool environment free of sunlight and moisture until needed — do not refrigerate.

Dosage for Tang or Decoction

To make a cup of tea use fifteen to thirty grams of herb to eight ounces of boiling water, steep and drink the warm strained decoction (tea), as needed.

Dosage for Powder

This formula should be taken twice daily. The powder can be taken in several different ways. Make a smoothie, by adding twenty to thirty grams of the powder to eight ounces of juice smoothie, mix well, and drink. If that is an issue we recommend adding twenty to thirty grams of the powdered herbs to 00-size capsules. For more detailed instructions, follow the step-by-step guide for preparing a smoothie or capsules discussed in Chapter Five.

* Dosage Note

The gram weight to be used in this formula is listed with a minimum/maximum range. This prescription should be prepared by using the lower dosage and only increase dosage to achieve stronger results when needed.

Herbal Ingredient

Grams	Chinese Herb	Botanical Name	Common Name
15-30*	Xi Fan Lian 西番莲	Passiflora Incarnata	Passionflower

DEMENTIA

Dementia is a general decline in mental ability whose most recognizable features are progressive intellectual impairment and memory loss. Possible causes include head injury, pernicious anemia, encephalitis, myxedema, syphilis, brain tumor, and alcoholism which can also be a contributing factor.

These reversible causes account for only about ten percent of dementia. The great majority of cases are a result of cerebrovascular disease such as stroke and Alzheimer's disease. The former can sometimes be helped by treatment of hypertension or heart disease when it is caused by the loss of blood supply to the brain due to narrowed or blocked arteries within the brain causing gradual deterioration. Alzheimer's disease which consists of a gradual loss of brain cells and shrinkage of brain substance, is irreversible.

The person with dementia may not remember recent events, may fail to grasp what is happening, and may become confused over days and dates.

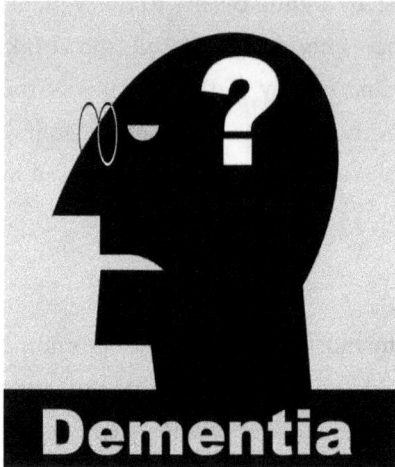
Dementia

These symptoms tend to come on gradually and may not be noticed right away. As dementia worsens, paranoia and depression with psychotic delusions may occur. In advanced stages, demented individuals usually lapse into a second childhood and require total nursing care including feeding, bathing and toilet, and aid with all physical activities.

Successful Chinese medical treatment depends on the use of herbal formulas that focus on relieving generalized weakness and fatigue, forgetfulness, being easily frightened, headache, vertigo, dizziness, tinnitus, and vascular dementia. The herbal formulas will address the underlying cause as well as treat the symptoms. Chinese herbs can certainly provide relief from the symptoms of dementia and improve the user's quality of life; however, it is advisable that the patient discontinue the use of alcohol.

All of the herbal prescriptions that follow can be effectively used to treat dementia. For each prescription, I have provided processing instructions and the prescription's therapeutic action.

RAW HERB FORMULAS
Shu Di Huang Yin Zi
Rehmannia Decoction

Therapeutic Actions
This prescription is used to treat dementia; it relieves the symptoms associated with dementia, including generalized weakness, fatigue, forgetfulness, and being easily frightened.

Preparation

Traditionally, this formula was used in the raw form to prepare a decoction; however, for those who have not developed the taste for harsh teas, we suggest the user have the ingredients ground into a fine powder by his/ her herb supplier, and then store the powder in a brown or amber glass bottle with a lid. Store it in a cool environment free of sunlight and moisture until needed — do not refrigerate.

Dosage for Tang or Decoction

Drink four ounces of the warm strained decoction (tea), three times during the day as needed.

Dosage for Powder

This formula should be taken twice daily. The powder can be taken in several different ways. Make a smoothie, by adding twenty to thirty grams of the powder to eight ounces of juice smoothie, mix well, and drink. If that is an issue we recommend adding twenty to thirty grams of the powdered herbs to 00-size capsules. For more detailed instructions, follow the step-by-step guide for preparing a smoothie or capsules discussed in Chapter Five.

Herbal Ingredients

Grams	Chinese Herb	Botanical Name	Common Name
9	Ba Ji Tian 巴戟天	*Morinda Officinalis*	Morinda Root
6	Fu Ling 茯苓	*Poria Cocos*	Tuckahoe
6	Fu Zi 附子	*Aconditum*	Aconite
6	Mai Men Dong 麦冬	*Ophiopogon*	Winter Wheat
9	Rou Cong Rong 肉苁蓉	*Cistanche*	Cistanche Salsa
6	Rou Gui 肉桂	*Cinnamomum*	Cinnamon Bark
9	Shan Zhu Yu 山茱萸	*Corni Fructus*	Dogwood Fruit
6	Shi Chang Pu 石菖蒲	*Acori*	Acorus
9	Shi Hu 石斛	*Dendrobium*	Dendrobium
12	Shu Di Huang 熟地黃	*Rehmanniae Preparata*	Rehmannia Cooked
6	Wu Wei Zi 五味子	*Schisandra*	Schizandra
6	Yuan Zhi 遠志	*Polygala Tenuifolia*	Milkwort Root

Contraindications

Do not use if pregnant, do not mix with alcohol, and do not use this formula in cases of heat or energy rising to your head, such as dizziness, hypertensive, or lightheaded.

Gou Teng San

Uncaria Powder

Therapeutic Actions

This prescription is used to relieve the symptoms of dementia; including but not limited to headache, vertigo, dizziness, tinnitus, Alzheimer's disease and dementia, and is used to treat vascular dementia as well as the impairment of memory caused by aging.

Preparation and Dosage

Grind the herbal ingredients into a fine powder, and store the powder in a brown or amber glass bottle with a lid. Store it in a cool environment free of sunlight and moisture until needed — do not refrigerate. The powder can be used in several different ways. Make a tea by adding nine grams of the powder to eight ounces of boiling water, add in seven slices of fresh ginger, remove from the heat source and allow it to steep for fifteen minutes and drink. The powder can also be added to a smoothie, add nine grams of the powder to eight ounces of juice smoothie mix well and drink. The formula can also be put into 00-size capsules, add twenty to thirty grams of powder to three capsules, take three capsules daily. For more detailed instructions, follow the step-by-step guide for preparing a decoction, smoothie or capsules discussed in Chapter Five.

Herbal Ingredients

Grams	Chinese Herb	Botanical Name	Common Name
15	Ban Xia 半夏	*Pinellia Ternata*	Half Summer
15	Chen Pi 陳皮	*Citrus Reticulate*	Tangerine Peel
15	Fang Feng 防風	*Ledebouriellae*	Siler
15	Fu Ling 茯苓	*Poria Cocos*	Tuckahoe
15	Fu Shen 茯神	*Poriae*	Hoelen Center
15	Gou Teng 勾藤	*Uncaria*	Gambir
15	Ju Hua 菊花	*Chrysanthemum*	Chrysanthemum
15	Mai Men Dong 麦冬	*Ophiopogon*	Winter Wheat
15	Ren Shen 人參	*Panax Ginseng*	Ginseng
30	Shi Gao 生石膏	*Gypsum Fibrosum*	Gypsum
3	Zhi Gan Cao 甘草	*Glycyrrhizae*	Licorice

Tong Qiao Huo Xue Tang

Unblock the Orifices and Invigorate the Blood Decoction

Therapeutic Actions

This prescription is used to treat dementia; it relieves blood stagnation in the head and face as well as the symptoms of dementia including: headache, dizziness, ringing in the ears, poor hearing, hair loss and lack of appetite.

Preparation

Traditionally, this formula was used in the raw form to prepare a decoction; however, for those who have not developed the taste for harsh teas, we suggest the user have the ingredients ground into a fine powder by his/her herb supplier, and then store the powder in a brown or amber glass bottle with a lid. Store it in a cool environment free of sunlight and moisture until needed — do not refrigerate.

*Dosage Note

The gram weight to be used in this formula is listed with a minimum/maximum range. This prescription should be prepared by using the lower dosage and only increase dosage to achieve stronger results when needed.

*Preparation Notes

The herb She Xiang should not be cooked. Do not add it to the herbs being cooked until the end of the cooking process.

The herb Sheng Jiang or fresh ginger should not be cooked for longer than five minutes. Do not add it to the herbs being cooked until the last five minutes of preparation time.

Dosage for Tang or Decoction

Drink four ounces of the warm strained decoction (tea), three times during the day as needed.

Dosage for Powder

This formula should be taken twice daily. The powder can be used in several different ways. Make a smoothie, by adding twenty to thirty grams of the powder to eight ounces of juice smoothie, mix well, and drink. If that is an issue we recommend adding twenty to thirty grams of the powdered herbs to 00-size capsules. For more detailed instructions, follow the step-by-step guide for preparing a smoothie or capsules discussed in Chapter Five.

Herbal Ingredients

Grams	Chinese Herb	Botanical Name	Common Name
3	Chi Shao 赤芍	*Paeonia Veitchii*	Red Peony
3	Chuan Xiong 川芎	*Ligusticum*	Cnidium
7 Pieces	Da Zao 大棗	*Ziziphus Jujuba*	Jujube
9	Hong Hua 紅花	*Carthamus*	Carthamus
3-6*	Lao Cong Bai 葱白	*Allium Fistulosum*	Scallion Sliced
0.15 Vial	She Xiang* 麝香	*Moschus Berezovskii*	Musk
9	Sheng Jiang* 生姜	*Zingiber Officinale*	Ginger Sliced
9	Tao Ren 桃仁	*Prunus Persica*	Peach Seed

Processing Note

The original prescription of this formula includes the herb She Xiang which is a derivative of an endangered species and I do not recommend that this herb should be used. I suggest that you replace it with an herbal substitute that has similar medical properties.

PATENT HERB FORMULA
Yin Xing Ye
Gingko Leaf Capsules

Therapeutic Actions

This patent formula is used to treat dementia; it invigorates the blood and nourishes the brain. It is used to enhance memory, concentration, and delay the effects of aging. This formula is useful for cerebral vascular insufficiency and headache.

Packaged

In bottle of one hundred capsules.

Dosage

Take one to two capsules, twice per day.

❋

DEPRESSION

People who suffer from depression make up approximately ten to fifteen percent of the U.S. population; which is why depression is considered the most common serious psychiatric illness in our country. Excessive use of drugs and/or alcohol can cause anxiety and depression, with incidents of suicide attempts and actual suicide being much higher among substance abusers. Those who suffer from this disorder experience feelings of sadness, hopelessness, pessimism, and a general loss of interest in life. Symptoms vary with the severity of the illness. In persons with mild depression, the main symptoms are anxiety and mood swings. Sufferers of this psychiatric disorder have also been known to have fits of crying for no apparent reason.

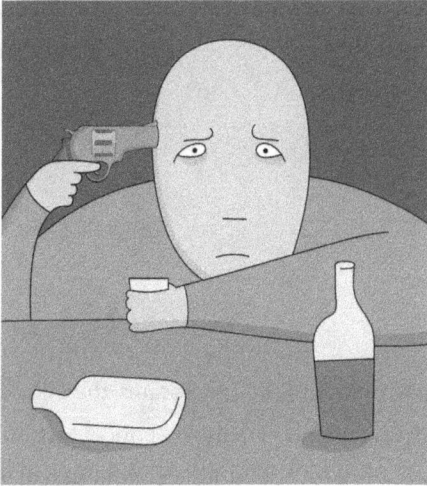

A person with more severe depression may suffer from loss of appetite, difficulty sleeping, loss of interest and enjoyment in social activities, feelings of tiredness and loss of concentration. In some cases, the opposite occurs and the person becomes extremely anxious and agitated. Severely depressed people may have thoughts of death and/or suicide, and feelings of guilt or worthlessness.

In extreme cases they may have hallucinations or delusions (believing, for example that someone is trying to poison them).

Although true depressive illness usually has no single obvious cause, it may be triggered by certain physical illnesses such as stroke, hepatitis, hormonal disorders such as hypothyroidism, or by hormonal changes that occur after childbirth; in that case, it is known as postpartum depression.

Depression appears to be more common in women, with approximately one in six seeking help for depression at some time in their lives as opposed to only one in nine men.

Depression can be successfully treated using Chinese herbal medicine; by consuming formulas that focus on relieving anxiety, depression, sadness, mood-swings, pain, hopelessness, and a general disinterest in life. In order for the treatment to be effective, complete abstinence from alcohol and/or drugs is recommended.

All of the herbal prescriptions that follow can be effectively used to treat depression. For each prescription, I will provide its unique processing instructions and therapeutic action.

RAW HERB FORMULAS
Ban Xia Hou Po Tang
Pinellia and Magnolia Bark Decoction

Therapeutic Actions
This prescription is used to treat depression as well as nervousness, stress, and panic disorder.

Preparation
Traditionally, this formula was used in the raw form to prepare a decoction; however, for those who have not developed the taste for harsh teas, we suggest the user have the ingredients ground into a fine powder by his/her herb supplier, and then store the powder in a brown or amber glass bottle with a lid. Store it in a cool environment free of sunlight and moisture until needed — do not refrigerate.

*Preparation Note
The herb Sheng Jiang or fresh ginger should not be cooked for longer than five minutes. Do not add it to the herbs being cooked until the last five minutes of preparation time.

Dosage for Tang or Decoction
Drink four ounces of the warm strained decoction (tea), three times during the day and once at night, as needed.

Dosage for Powder
This formula should be taken three times daily. The powder can be used in several different ways. Make a smoothie, by adding twenty to thirty grams of the powder to four-eight ounces of juice smoothie, mix well, and drink. If that is an issue we recommend adding twenty to thirty grams of the powdered herbs to 00-size capsules. For more detailed instructions, follow the step-by-step guide for preparing a smoothie or capsules discussed in Chapter Five.

Herbal Ingredients

Grams	Chinese Herb	Botanical Name	Common Name
12	Ban Xia 半夏	*Pinellia Ternata*	Half Summer
12	Fu Ling 茯苓	*Poria Cocos*	Tuckahoe
9	Hou Po 厚朴	*Magnolia Officinalis*	Magnolia Bark
15	Sheng Jiang* 生姜	*Zingiber Officinale*	Ginger Sliced
6	Zi Su Ye 紫蘇	*Perilla Frutescens*	Perilla Leaf

Ban Xia Xie Xin Tang

Pinellia Decoction to Drain the Epigastrium

Therapeutic Actions

This prescription is used to treat depression associated with addiction, as well as hepatitis and liver cirrhosis; it is also effective for acid reflux and diarrhea.

Preparation

Traditionally, this formula was used in the raw form to prepare a decoction; however, for those who have not developed the taste for harsh teas, we suggest the user have the ingredients ground into a fine powder by his/her herb supplier, and then store the powder in a brown or amber glass bottle with a lid. Store it in a cool environment free of sunlight and moisture until needed — do not refrigerate.

Dosage for Tang or Decoction

Drink eight ounces of the warm strained decoction (tea), once a day as needed.

Dosage for Powder

This formula should be taken twice daily. The powder can be used in several different ways. Make a smoothie, by adding twenty to thirty grams of the powder to eight ounces of juice smoothie, mix well, and drink. If that is an issue we recommend adding twenty to thirty grams of the powdered herbs to 00-size capsules. For more detailed instructions, follow the step-by-step guide for preparing a smoothie or capsules discussed in Chapter Five.

Herbal Ingredients

Grams	Chinese Herb	Botanical Name	Common Name
9	Ban Xia 半夏	*Pinellia Ternata*	Half Summer
4 Pieces	Da Zao 大棗	*Ziziphus Jujuba*	Jujube
9	Gan Jiang 乾薑	*Zingiber Officinale*	Ginger, Dried
3	Huang Lian 黃連	*Coptis*	Coptis Root
9	Huang Qin 黃芩	*Schutellaria*	Baikal Skullcap
9	Ren Shen 人參	*Ginseng*	Ginseng
6	Zhi Gan Cao 甘草	*Glycyrrhizae*	Licorice

Contraindication

Do not use this formula when bloated or for those suffering from nausea or vomiting.

Xiao Jian Zhong Tang

Minor Construct the Middle Decoction

Therapeutic Actions

This prescription is used to treat depression; it relieves depression and improves the mood and is used for relief from severe depression. It is also very effective for stimulating appetite and treating malnutrition.

Preparation

Traditionally, this formula was used in the raw form to prepare a decoction; however, for those who have not developed the taste for harsh teas, we suggest the user have the ingredients ground into a fine powder by his/her herb supplier, and then store the powder in a brown or amber glass bottle with a lid. Store it in a cool environment free of sunlight and moisture until needed — do not refrigerate.

*Preparation Notes

The herb Yi Tang should not be cooked. Only after the cooking process is completed should you add this herb to the pot, and stir the brew to allow it to dissolve. Then strain off the herbs. The herb Sheng Jiang or fresh ginger should not be cooked for longer than five minutes. Do not add it to the herbs being cooked until the last five minutes of preparation time.

Dosage for Tang or Decoction
Drink eight ounces of the warm strained decoction (tea), three times a day as needed.

Dosage for Powder
This formula should be taken twice daily. The powder can be used in several different ways. Make a smoothie, by adding twenty to thirty grams of the powder to eight ounces of juice smoothie, mix well, and drink. If that is an issue we recommend adding twenty to thirty grams of the powdered herbs to 00-size capsules. For more detailed instructions, follow the step-by-step guide for preparing a smoothie or capsules discussed in Chapter Five.

Herbal Ingredients

Grams	Chinese Herb	Botanical Name	Common Name
18	Bai Shao 白芍	*Paeonia*	White Peony
4 Pieces	Da Zao 大棗	*Ziziphus Jujuba*	Jujube
9	Gui Zhi 桂枝	*Cinnamomum*	Cinnamon Twigs
9	Sheng Jiang* 生姜	*Zingiber Officinale*	Ginger, Sliced
30	Yi Tang★ 饴糖	*Sacchrum Granorum*	Maltose
6	Zhi Gan Cao 甘草	*Glycyrrhizae*	Licorice

Contraindication
This formula should not be used by patients who have intestinal parasites.

PATENT HERB FORMULAS
An Shui Wan Teapills
Peaceful Sleep Pills

Therapeutic Actions
This patent formula is used to treat depression, anxiety disorders, and panic attacks with or without insomnia, restlessness, palpitations, vivid dreams and fatigue.

Cautions
Do not use if pregnant. Overdosing may cause drowsiness.

Packaged
In bottle of two hundred pills.

Dosage
Take two pills as needed; dosage can be increased to three pills three times daily.

Gan Mai Da Zao Wan
Glycyrrhiza, Triticum, Jujube Pills

Therapeutic Actions
This patent formula is used to treat depression with restless sleep, and anxiety, excessive worrying, crying, insomnia, clouded mind, or vivid dreaming.

Packaged
In bottle of two hundred pills.

Dosage
Take eight pills three times daily; dosage can be increased to twelve pills if needed.

DIABETES MELLITUS

In African American communities throughout the U.S. approximately one out of every six people are affected by diabetes that is a result of the pancreas producing an insufficient amount of insulin (the hormone responsible for the absorption of glucose) or no insulin at all. Commonly referred to in black vernacular as "sugar," the disease's clinical name is diabetes mellitus.

COMMON DIABETES SYMPTOMS

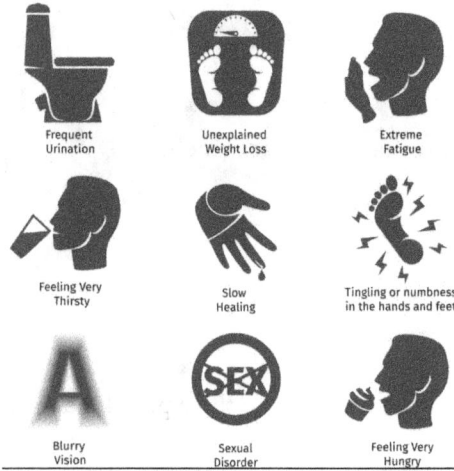

Frequent Urination

Unexplained Weight Loss

Extreme Fatigue

Feeling Very Thirsty

Slow Healing

Tingling or numbness in the hands and feet

Blurry Vision

Sexual Disorder

Feeling Very Hungry

When an insufficient amount of insulin is produced to absorb the glucose, the level of glucose in the blood becomes abnormally high, causing symptoms such as: constant thirst, frequent urination and hunger. The body's inability to store or use glucose causes weight loss and fatigue. Diabetes mellitus also impairs the body's ability to metabolize lipids as well as accelerating the degeneration of the small blood vessels which impedes blood circulation to the extremities (hands and feet).

While no one would argue against the fact that obesity plays a major role in the disease, illnesses such as pancreatitis can aggravate the onset of diabetes. In fact, long-term and excessive alcohol consumption's harmful effect on the pancreas—which often hinders the gland's ability to produce sufficient amounts of the enzyme insulin—is in a large number of cases, the underlying cause that triggers diabetes.

There are two main types of diabetes mellitus, insulin dependent (type 1) the more severe form, and the non-insulin dependent (type 2).

Because the pancreas does produce some insulin in non-insulin dependent (type 2) diabetes, the disorder can often be controlled by dietary means alone by regulating the intake of carbohydrates and alcohol consumption. This not only lowers the blood glucose levels, it also reduces weight. If diet fails to lower the glucose level sufficiently, hypoglycemic tablets (oral anti-diabetic drugs that stimulate the pancreas to produce more insulin) may be prescribed.

People with insulin dependent (type 1) diabetes must inject themselves one to four times a day, in order to avoid marked fluctuations in the glucose levels in the blood.

Disturbances in the delicate balance between insulin and glucose intake can result in hyperglycemia (too much glucose in the blood) or hypoglycemia (too little glucose), which can lead to weakness, confusion, dizziness, sweating, unconsciousness and seizures. To prevent this, diabetics are advised to regularly monitor their blood and urine glucose level.

Chinese herbs can successfully treat diabetes mellitus, by lowering blood sugar levels and relieving the common symptoms; however, I would be remiss if I did not recommend that the patient discontinue use of alcohol.

Note

When taking Chinese herbal formulas that treat diabetes the user should closely monitor his/her blood glucose level. It is also wise to discuss your plans to use Chinese herbal formulas with your primary care physician and together you can monitor your diabetes and maintain a healthy glucose level.

All of the herbal prescriptions that follow can be effectively used to treat diabetes. For each prescription I will provide its unique processing instructions and therapeutic action.

RAW HERB FORMULAS
Liu Wei Di Huang
Six Ingredient Pill with Rehmannia

Therapeutic Actions
This formula is used to treat the symptoms of diabetes; primarily it will

alleviate thirst, reduce urinary frequency and blood glucose levels, eliminate night sweats, alleviate dizziness, ringing in the ears, and blurred vision.

Preparation

Traditionally, this formula was used in the raw form to prepare a decoction; however, for those who have not developed the taste for harsh teas, we suggest the user have the ingredients ground into a fine powder by his/her herb supplier, and then store the powder in a brown or amber glass bottle with a lid. Store it in a cool environment free of sunlight and moisture until needed — do not refrigerate.

Dosage for Tang or Decoction

Drink four ounces of the warm strained decoction (tea), three times a day as needed.

Dosage for Powder

This formula should be taken twice daily. The powder can be used in several different ways. Make a smoothie, by adding twenty to thirty grams of the powder to eight ounces of juice smoothie, mix well, and drink. If that is an issue we recommend adding twenty to thirty grams of the powdered herbs to 00-size capsules. For more detailed instructions, follow the step-by-step guide for preparing a smoothie or capsules discussed in Chapter Five.

Herbal Ingredients

Grams	Chinese Herb	Botanical Name	Common Name
9	Fu Ling 茯苓	*Poria Cocos*	Tuckahoe
9	Mu Dan Pi 牡丹皮	*Paeonia Suffruticosa*	Tree Peony Bark
12	Shan Yao 山药	*Dioscorea Opposite*	Yam
12	Shan Zhu Yu 山茱萸	*Corni Fructus*	Dogwood Fruit
24	Shu Di Huang 熟地黃	*Rehmanniae Preparata*	Rehmannia Cooked
9	Ze Xie 澤瀉	*Alisma Orientalis*	Water Plantain

Contraindication

Do not use this prescription if you suffer from low blood sugar levels.

Long Dan Xie Gan Tang

Gentiana Decoction to Drain the Liver

Therapeutic Actions

This formula is used to treat the symptoms of diabetes; characterized by obesity, and elevated cholesterol and/or triglyceride levels.

Preparation

Traditionally, this formula was used in the raw form to prepare a decoction; however, for those who have not developed the taste for harsh teas, we suggest the user have the ingredients ground into a fine powder by his/her herb supplier, and then store the powder in a brown or amber glass bottle with a lid. Store it in a cool environment free of sunlight and moisture until needed — do not refrigerate.

Dosage for Tang or Decoction

Drink four ounces of the warm strained decoction (tea), three times a day as needed.

Dosage for Powder

This formula should be taken twice daily. The powder can be used in several different ways. Make a smoothie, by adding twenty to thirty grams of the powder to eight ounces of juice smoothie, mix well, and drink. If that is an issue we recommend adding twenty to thirty grams of the powdered herbs to 00-size capsules. For more detailed instructions, follow the step-by-step guide for preparing a smoothie or capsules discussed in Chapter Five.

Herbal Ingredients

Grams	Chinese Herb	Botanical Name	Common Name
6	Chai Hu 柴胡	*Bupleurum*	Bupleurum
9	Che Qian Zi 車前子	*Plantago*	Plantago Seed
9	Chuan Mu Tong 川木通	*Clematis*	Clematis
3	Dang Gui 當歸	*Angelica*	Angelica
6	Gan Cao 甘草	*Glycyrrhiza*	Licorice
9	Huang Qin 黃芩	*Schutellaria*	Baikal Skullcap
6	Long Dan 龙胆	*Gentiana Scabra*	Gentian
9	Shu Di Huang 熟地黃	*Rehmanniae Preparata*	Rehmannia Cooked
12	Ze Xie 澤瀉	*Alisma Orientalis*	Water Plantain
9	Zhi Zi 栀子	Gardenia	Gardenia

Contraindication

This formula should not be used for those with blood deficiencies.

Yu Ye Tang

Jade Fluid Decoction

Therapeutic Actions

This formula is used to treat the symptoms of diabetes; primarily it will alleviate thirst, and moistens dryness.

Preparation

Traditionally, this formula was used in the raw form to prepare a decoction; however, for those who have not developed the taste for harsh teas, we suggest the user have the ingredients ground into a fine powder by his/ her herb supplier, and then store the powder in a brown or amber glass bottle with a lid. Store it in a cool environment free of sunlight and moisture until needed — do not refrigerate.

Dosage for Tang or Decoction

Drink four ounces of the warm strained decoction (tea), three times a day as needed.

Dosage for Powder

This formula should be taken twice daily. The powder can be used in several different ways. Make a smoothie, by adding twenty to thirty grams of the powder to eight ounces of juice smoothie, mix well, and drink. If that is an issue we recommend adding twenty to thirty grams of the powdered herbs to 00-size capsules. For more detailed instructions, follow the step-by-step guide for preparing a smoothie or capsules discussed in Chapter Five.

Herbal Ingredients

Grams	Chinese Herb	Botanical Name	Common Name
4.5	Ge Gen 葛根	*Puerariae*	Kudzu
15	Huang Qi 黄芪	*Astragalus*	Milkvetch Root
6	Ji Nei Jin 鸡内金	*Gallus*	Chicken Gizzard
30	Shan Yao 山药	*Dioscorea Opposite*	Yam
9	Tian Hua Fen 天花粉	*Trichosanthes*	Trichosanthes
9	Wu Wei Zi 五味子	*Schisandra*	Schizandra
18	Zhi Mu 知母	*Anemarrhena*	Anemarrhena

Contraindication

Do not use this prescription if you suffer from low blood sugar level.

PATENT HERB FORMULAS
Ku Qiao Mai

Tartarian Buckwheat

Therapeutic Actions

This patent formula is used to treat diabetes; it strengthens blood vessels benefiting blood pressure and improving circulation to the eyes, and improves glucose metabolism.

Packaged

In bottle of one hundred capsules.

Dosage

Take one capsule two times daily.

Yu Quan Wan

Jade Spring Pills

Therapeutic Actions

This patent formula is used to treat diabetes with symptoms of thirst, frequent urination, excessive hunger, weight loss, fatigue, and turbid urine.

Cautions

Use prohibited during pregnancy. Do not use with pharmaceutical glybenzycyclamide.

Packaged

In bottle of two hundred pills.

Dosage

Take eight pills three times daily; dosage can be increased to twelve pills if needed.

🍁

DIARRHEA

Increased fluidity, frequency, or volume of bowel movements, compared to the usual pattern for a particular person. Diarrhea itself is not a disorder but is a symptom of an underlying problem. The most frequent cause for acute diarrhea, commonly referred to as the runs, is food poisoning, drug toxicity, food allergies and excess alcohol consumption.

Chronic diarrhea, which takes the form of repeated attacks, is usually caused by Crohn's disease, ulcerative colitis, diverticular disease, cancer of the large intestine and irritable bowel syndrome. In all of these conditions with the exception of irritable bowel syndrome, there may be blood in the feces.

The water and electrolytes lost during a severe attack of diarrhea need to be replaced to avoid dehydration. Diarrhea that recurs, persists for more than a week or is accompanied by blood in the bowel movements requires investigation to determine the underlying cause.

Successful Chinese herbal treatment focuses on relieving bloating, cramping, vomiting, loose stools and nausea. The herbs in these formulas will address the underlying cause, and treat the symptoms. The user is encouraged to discontinue use of alcohol and/or drugs. If this is carried out, full recovery is possible, without permanent damage to the intestine or colon.

All of the herbal prescriptions that follow can be effectively used to treat diarrhea. For each prescription, I will provide its unique processing instructions and therapeutic action.

RAW HERB FORMULA
Ban Xia Xie Xin Tang
Pinellia Decoction to Drain the Epigastrium

Therapeutic Actions
This prescription is used to treat diarrhea; as well as hepatitis, liver cirrhosis, acid reflux, and depression.

Preparation
Traditionally, this formula was used in the raw form to prepare a decoction; however, for those who have not developed the taste for harsh teas, we suggest the user have the ingredients ground into a fine powder by his/ her herb supplier, and then store the powder in a brown or amber glass bottle with a lid. Store it in a cool environment free of sunlight and moisture until needed — do not refrigerate.

Dosage for Tang or Decoction

Drink eight ounces of the warm strained decoction (tea), once a day as needed.

Dosage for Powder

This formula should be taken once daily. The powder can be used in several different ways. Make a smoothie, by adding twenty to thirty grams of the powder to eight ounces of juice smoothie, mix well, and drink. If that is an issue we recommend adding twenty to thirty grams of the powdered herbs to 00-size capsules. For more detailed instructions, follow the step-by-step guide for preparing a smoothie or capsules discussed in Chapter Five.

Herbal Ingredients

Grams	Chinese Herb	Botanical Name	Common Name
9	Ban Xia 半夏	*Pinellia Ternata*	Half Summer
4 Pieces	Da Zao 大棗	*Ziziphus Jujuba*	Jujube
9	Gan Jiang 乾薑	*Zingiber Officinale*	Ginger, Dried
3	Huang Lian 黃連	*Coptis*	Coptis Root
9	Huang Qin 黃芩	*Schutellaria*	Baikal Skullcap
9	Ren Shen 人参	*Ginseng*	Ginseng
6	Zhi Gan Cao 甘草	*Glycyrrhizae*	Licorice

PATENT HERB FORMULAS

Bao Ji Wan

Po Chi Pills

Therapeutic Actions

This patent formula is used to treat diarrhea, and the symptoms of a hangover or heartburn; including nausea, bloating, stomach cramping, and vomiting.

Packaged

In box containing ten vials of pills.

Dosage

Take the full contents of one-two vials up to three times daily.

Bu Zhong Yi Qi Tang

Tonify Center, Increase Chi Pills, Central Chi Pills

Therapeutic Actions

This patent formula is used to treat chronic diarrhea associated with cirrhosis and hepatitis; it relieves poor digestion with loose stools, chronic diarrhea, and flatulence.

Packaged

In bottle of two hundred pills.

Dosage

Take eight pills, three times per day. Dosage can be increase to twelve pills, if needed.

🍁

ENLARGED LIVER

aka Fatty Liver

The effect of alcohol on the liver is direct and toxic. The job of breaking down alcohol in the body—which is the function of the liver—is the reason that it is the primary site of some of the most serious alcohol-related disorders.

Heading the list of liver ailments frequently seen in cases of alcohol abuse is enlargement of the liver. This preliminary damage to one of the body's most vital organs often leads to diseases like hepatitis and cirrhosis.

Sometimes referred to as fatty liver disease, quite often there are no obvious symptoms, but an enlarged liver may be noted during a physical examination. In other patients there may be pain in the upper right side of the abdomen, developing a barrel-like chest, and/or jaundice (the skin eyes and other tissue take on a yellowish hue).

Diagnosis of an enlarged liver is made by obtaining a sample of liver tissue and noting the abnormal presence of fatty deposits.

Successful Chinese medical treatment depends on the use of herbal formulas that focus on detoxifying the organ along with addressing the underlying cause, and discontinuing the use of alcohol. If this is carried out, full recovery is possible—without permanent damage to the organ.

The herbal prescriptions that follow can be effectively used to treat enlarged liver or fatty liver. For each prescription, I will provide its unique processing instructions and therapeutic action.

RAW HERB FORMULAS
Da Chai Hu Tang
Major Bupleurum Decoction

Therapeutic Actions
This formula is used to treat the symptoms of enlarged liver or fatty liver; including pain in the upper right side of the abdomen, developing a barrel-like chest, and/or jaundice.

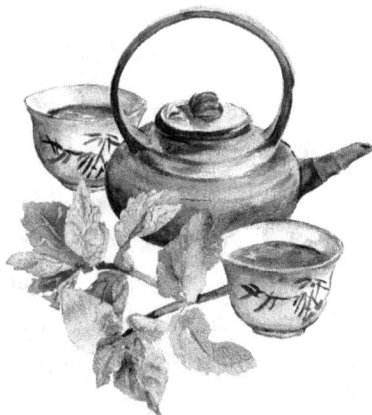

Preparation
Traditionally, this formula was used in the raw form to prepare a decoction; however, for those who have not developed the taste for harsh teas, we suggest the user have the ingredients ground into a fine powder by his/her herb supplier,

and then store the powder in a brown or amber glass bottle with a lid. Store it in a cool environment free of sunlight and moisture until needed — do not refrigerate.

*Preparation Note

The herb Sheng Jiang or fresh ginger should not be cooked for longer than five minutes. Do not add it to the herbs being cooked until the last five minutes of preparation time.

Dosage for Tang or Decoction

Drink eight ounces of warm strained decoction, once daily.

Dosage for Powder

This formula should be taken once daily. The powder can be used in several different ways. Make a smoothie, by adding twenty to thirty grams of the powder to eight ounces of juice smoothie, mix well, and drink. If that is an issue we recommend adding twenty to thirty grams of the powdered herbs to 00-size capsules. For more detailed instructions, follow the step-by-step guide for preparing a smoothie or capsules discussed in Chapter Five.

Herbal Ingredients

Grams	Chinese Herb	Botanical Name	Common Name
9	Bai Shao 白芍	*Paeonia*	White Peony
9	Ban Xia 半夏	*Pinellia Ternata*	Half Summer
15	Chai Hu 柴胡	*Bupleurum*	Bupleurum
6	Da Huang 大黃	*Rheum Palmatum*	Rhubarb Root
4 Pieces	Da Zao 大棗	*Ziziphus Jujuba*	Jujube
9	Huang Qin 黃芩	*Schutellaria*	Baikal Skullcap
15	Sheng Jiang* 生姜	*Zingiber Officinale*	Ginger, Sliced
9	Zhi Shi 炒枳實	*Citrus Aurantium*	Bitter Orange

Contraindication

Avoid eating cold, raw or pungent or spicy food while taking this formula.

Chai Ling Tang

Bupleurum and Poria Decoction

Therapeutic Actions

This formula is used to treat the symptoms of enlarged liver or fatty liver; including pain in the upper right side of the abdomen, developing a barrel-like chest, and/or jaundice.

Preparation

Traditionally, this formula was used in the raw form to prepare a decoction; however, for those who have not developed the taste for harsh teas, we suggest the user have the ingredients ground into a fine powder by his/ her herb supplier, and then store the powder in a brown or amber glass bottle with a lid. Store it in a cool environment free of sunlight and moisture until needed — do not refrigerate.

*Preparation Note

The herb Sheng Jiang or fresh ginger should not be cooked for longer than five minutes. Do not add it to the herbs being cooked until the last five minutes of preparation time.

Dosage for Tang or Decoction

Drink four to eight ounces of the warm strained decoction once daily.

Dosage for Powder

This formula should be taken once daily. The powder can be used in several different ways. Make a smoothie, by adding twenty to thirty grams of the powder to eight ounces of juice smoothie, mix well, and drink. If that is an issue we recommend adding twenty to thirty grams of the powdered herbs to 00-size capsules. For more detailed instructions, follow the step-by-step guide for preparing a smoothie or capsules discussed in Chapter Five.

Herbal Ingredients

Grams	Chinese Herb	Botanical Name	Common Name
9	Bai Zhu 白术	*Atractylodes*	Atractylodes
9	Ban Xia 半夏	*Pinellia Ternata*	Half Summer
12	Chai Hu 柴胡	*Bupleurum*	Bupleurum
9	Fu Ling 茯苓	*Poria Cocos*	Tuckahoe
6	Gui Zhi 桂枝	*Cinnamomum*	Cinnamon Twigs
9	Huang Qin 黃芩	*Schutellaria*	Baikal Skullcap
6	Ren Shen 人参	*Ginseng*	Ginseng
9	Sheng Jiang* 生姜	*Zingiber Officinale*	Ginger, Sliced
15	Ze Xie 澤瀉	*Alisma Orientalis*	Water Plantain
5	Zhi Gan Cao 甘草	*Glycyrrhizae*	Licorice
9	Zhu Ling 豬苓	*Polyporus*	Polyporus

Contraindication
Avoid eating cold, raw or pungent or spicy food while taking this formula.

Yi Guan Jian
Linking Decoction

Therapeutic Actions
This formula can be used during to treat the symptoms of enlarged liver or fatty liver, it is very useful when there is chest pain, abdominal distention (bloated stomach), dry mouth, acid regurgitation, and loss of weight, and it is extremely useful in the early stages of cirrhosis.

Preparation
Traditionally, this formula was used in the raw form to prepare a decoction; however, for those who have not developed the taste for harsh teas, we suggest the user have the ingredients ground into a fine powder by his/

her herb supplier, and then store the powder in a brown or amber glass bottle with a lid. Store it in a cool environment free of sunlight and moisture until needed — do not refrigerate.

*Dosage Note

The gram weight to be used in this formula is listed with a minimum/maximum range. This prescription should be prepared by using the lower dosage and only increase dosage to achieve stronger results when needed.

Dosage for Tang or Decoction

Drink four to eight ounces of the warm strained decoction (tea), three times during the day as needed.

Dosage for Powder

This formula should be taken twice daily. The powder can be used in several different ways. Make a smoothie, by adding twenty to thirty grams of the powder to eight ounces of juice smoothie, mix well, and drink. If that is an issue we recommend adding twenty to thirty grams of the powdered herbs to 00-size capsules. For more detailed instructions, follow the step-by-step guide for preparing a smoothie or capsules discussed in Chapter Five.

Herbal Ingredients

Grams	Chinese Herb	Botanical Name	Common Name
9	Bei Sha Shen 北沙蔘	*Glehniae*	Glehnia
4.5	Chuan Lian Zi 川楝子	*Melia Toosendan*	Chinaberry Fruit
9	Dang Gui 當歸	*Angelica*	Angelica
9-18*	Gou Qi Zi 枸杞子	*Lycii Fructus*	Wolfberry
9	Mai Men Dong 麦冬	*Ophiopogon*	Winter Wheat
18-45*	Sheng Di Huang 生地黃	*Rehmannia*	Rehmannia, Dried

PATENT HERB FORMULA
Yi Guan Jian Wan
Linking Decoction Pills

Therapeutic Actions
This patent formula is used to treat enlarged liver, fatty liver or chronic hepatitis; symptoms include distention, nausea, pain, acid regurgitation, and belching.

Caution
Do not use this formula if you are producing phlegm and damp (mucus).

Packaged
In bottle of two hundred pills.

Dosage
Take eight pills three times daily (dosage can be increased to twelve pills if needed).

❋

GASTRITIS

Practically everyone who has the misfortune to suffer from gastritis will agree that it is one of the worse stomachaches that they have ever experienced! What is considered by many of its unfortunate sufferers to be the "mother of all bellyaches" is caused by digestive enzymes irritating the stomach and inflaming the stomach-wall by altering its mucous lining.

Gastritis produces many of the same symptoms as a gastric ulcer, with which it may be confused. Typical symptoms are: discomfort in the upper abdomen, which is often aggravated by eating, nausea and vomiting. Excessive use of alcohol can be a contributing factor or cause of this disease.

Gastritis can be acute, occurring as a sudden attack, or chronic, developing gradually over a longer period of time. Acute gastritis may cause erosions in the stomach lining that bleed easily. In the chronic form, blood may ooze continually from the stomach lining. Bleeding from the stomach lining causes the feces to appear black. Slow continual bleeding, which occurs in the chronic form of the disease, can also cause iron-deficiency anemia with symptoms such as parlor (pale complexion), fatigue, and shortness of breath.

If Western medicine's analgesics are taken for pain relief, a person suffering from gastritis should take acetaminophen rather than aspirin, and avoid alcohol and all forms of smoking (cigarette, cigars, pipe, crack, marijuana, e-cigarettes, etc.) which can intensify the symptoms.

The Chinese herbal formulas used to treat gastritis contain ingredients that eliminate stomach heat, arrest bleeding, stop vomiting, and relieve nausea. Once the stomach lining has healed, which normally takes from one to three weeks, depending on the severity of the inflammation, under normal circumstances the patient should be able to look forward to complete recovery.

All of the herbal prescriptions that follow can be effectively used to treat gastritis. For each prescription, I will provide its unique processing instructions and therapeutic action.

RAW HERB FORMULAS
Da Jian Zhong Tang
Major Construct the Middle Decoction

Therapeutic Actions
This prescription is used to treat the symptoms of gastritis as well as gastric and duodenal ulcers.

Preparation
Traditionally, this formula was used in the raw form to prepare a decoction; however, for those who have not developed the taste for harsh teas, we suggest the user have the ingredients ground into a fine powder by his/ her herb supplier, and then store the powder in a brown or amber glass

bottle with a lid. Store it in a cool environment free of sunlight and moisture until needed — do not refrigerate.

*Preparation Note

The herb Yi Tang should not be cooked. Only after the cooking process is completed should you add this herb to the pot, and stir the brew to allow it to dissolve. Then strain off the herbs.

Dosage for Tang or Decoction

Drink four to eight ounces of the warm strained decoction (tea), three times during the day as needed.

Dosage for Powder

This formula should be taken twice daily. The powder can be used in several different ways. Make a smoothie, by adding twenty to thirty grams of the powder to eight ounces of juice smoothie, mix well, and drink. If that is an issue we recommend adding twenty to thirty grams of the powdered herbs to 00-size capsules. For more detailed instructions, follow the step-by-step guide for preparing a smoothie or capsules discussed in Chapter Five.

Herbal Ingredients

Grams	Chinese Herb	Botanical Name	Common Name
4.5	Gan Jiang 乾薑	*Zingiber Officinale*	Ginger Dried
3	Hua Jiao 花椒	*Zanthoxylum*	Prickly Ash Pepper
6	Ren Shen 人参	*Ginseng*	Ginseng
3	Yi Tang* 饴糖	*Sacchrum Granorum*	Maltose

Ju Pi Zhu Ru Tang

Tangerine Peel and Bamboo Shavings Decoction

Therapeutic Actions

This prescription is used to treat the symptoms of gastritis; it stops vomiting, relieves nausea, alleviates thirst, and restores the appetite.

Preparation

Traditionally, this formula was used in the raw form to prepare a decoction; however, for those who have not developed the taste for harsh teas, we suggest the user have the ingredients ground into a fine powder by his/her herb supplier, and then store the powder in a brown or amber glass bottle with a lid. Store it in a cool environment free of sunlight and moisture until needed — do not refrigerate.

Dosage for Tang or Decoction

Drink four to eight ounces of the warm strained decoction (tea), once daily as needed.

Dosage for Powder

This formula should be taken once daily. The powder can be used in several different ways. Make a smoothie, by adding twenty to thirty grams of the powder to eight ounces of juice smoothie, mix well, and drink. If that is an issue we recommend adding twenty to thirty grams of the powdered herbs to 00-size capsules. For more detailed instructions, follow the step-by-step guide for preparing a smoothie or capsules discussed in Chapter Five.

Herbal Ingredients

Grams	Chinese Herb	Botanical Name	Common Name
30	Ban Xia 半夏	*Pinellia Ternata*	Half Summer
30	Chen Pi 陳皮	*Citrus Reticulate*	Tangerine Peel
30	Fu Ling 茯苓	*Poria Cocos*	Tuckahoe
30	Mai Men Dong 麦冬	*Ophiopogon*	Winter Wheat
30	Pi Pa Ye 枇杷叶	*Eriobotrya*	Loquat Leaf
15	Ren Shen 人参	*Ginseng*	Ginseng
15	Zhi Gan Cao 甘草	*Glycyrrhizae*	Licorice
30	Zhu Ru 竹茹	*Bambusa*	Bamboo Shavings

PATENT HERB FORMULAS
Wei Yao
707 Gastropathy Capsules

Therapeutic Actions
This patent formula is used to treat gastritis; it relieves excess stomach acid without bleeding, and can be used for inflammation of the stomach or intestinal lining.

Packaged
In bottle of forty two capsules.

Dosage
Take two to three capsules, three times daily.

Wei Te Ling Pills
204 Wei Te

Therapeutic Actions
This patent formula is used to treat gastritis; it relieves excess acid, prevents acid reflux, heartburn and epigastric pain. This formula can be used for treating gastro-esophageal reflux, acid regurgitation, as well as chronic and acute gastritis.

Packaged
In bottle of one hundred pills

Dosage
Take eight pills, one to two times daily as needed.

GONORRHEA

Gonorrhea is a sexually transmitted disease, also known as "the clap." Gonorrhea is caused by the bacterium Neisseria Gonorrhoeae, which is most frequently transmitted during sexual intercourse, including oral and anal sex.

Infection acquired through anal sex causes inflammation of the anus and/or rectum, and can result in pain and anal discharge in approximately ten percent of infected people. Oral sex with an infected person may lead to gonnococcal pharyngitis (soreness in the throat).

Babies exposed to the infection in the mother's reproductive tract during childbirth may acquire gonococcol ophthalmia, a severe inflammation affecting one or both eyes.

In men, symptoms usually include a urethral discharge and pain on urination. Approximately sixty percent of infected women have no symptoms; if symptoms are present, they usually consist of a vaginal discharge or a burning sensation when urinating.

As with all STD it is advisable to treat all sexual partners to avoid reinfection.

Successful Chinese medical treatment uses powerful herbal formulas that focus on treating the bacterial infection, relieving the symptoms of infection including abdominal pain, genital discomfort, discharge, itching, and lower back pain.

All of the herbal prescriptions that follow can be effectively used to treat gonorrhea. For each prescription, I will provide its unique processing instructions and therapeutic action.

RAW HERB FORMULAS
Ba Wei Dai Xia Fang
Eight-Ingredient Formula for Leukorrhea

Therapeutic Actions
This prescription is used to treat gonorrhea; it relieves infection

characterized by damp-heat in the lower Jiao (lower body); leukorrhea infection with yellow, white, or red discharge, generalized itching and discomfort in the genital region, abdominal pain, soreness of the lower back, and slight anemia. This formula is also very effective for acute or chronic leukorrhea, trichomoniasis, and uteritis.

Preparation

Traditionally, this formula was used in the raw form to prepare a decoction; however, for those who have not developed the taste for harsh teas, we suggest the user have the ingredients ground into a fine powder by his/her herb supplier, and then store the powder in a brown or amber glass bottle with a lid. Store it in a cool environment free of sunlight and moisture until needed — do not refrigerate.

Dosage for Tang or Decoction

Drink four ounces of the warm strained decoction (tea), three times during the day as needed.

Dosage for Powder

This formula should be taken twice daily. The powder can be used in several different ways. Make a smoothie, by adding twenty to thirty grams of the powder to eight ounces of juice smoothie, mix well, and drink. If that is an issue we recommend adding twenty to thirty grams of the powdered herbs to 00-size capsules. For more detailed instructions, follow the step-by-step guide for preparing a smoothie or capsules discussed in Chapter Five.

Notes

This treatment is more effective when it's combined with the patent pill formula Long Dan Xie Gan Wan. As with all STD it is advisable to treat all sexual partners to avoid reinfection.

Herbal Ingredients

Grams	Chinese Herb	Botanical Name	Common Name
2	Chen Pi 陳皮	*Citrus Reticulate*	Tangerine Peel
3	Chuan Mu Tong 川木通	*Clematis Armandii*	Clematis
3	Chuan Xiong 川芎	*Ligusticum*	Cnidium
0.5	Da Huang 大黃	*Rheum Palmatum*	Rhubarb Root
5	Dang Gui 當歸	*Angelica*	Angelica
3	Fu Ling 茯苓	*Poria Cocos*	Tuckahoe
2	Jin Yin Hua 金银花	*Lonicera*	Honeysuckle
4	Tu Fu Ling 土茯苓	*Smilax Glabra*	Smilax

Dang Gui Nian Tong Tang

Tangkuei Decoction to Lift the Pain

Therapeutic Actions

This formula is used to treat gonorrhea; it will heal the symptoms of dermatitis and genital itching.

Preparation

Traditionally, this formula was used in the raw form to prepare a decoction; however, for those who have not developed the taste for harsh teas, we suggest the user have the ingredients ground into a fine powder by his/her herb supplier, and then store the powder in a brown or amber glass bottle with a lid. Store it in a cool environment free of sunlight and moisture until needed — do not refrigerate

Dosage for Tang or Decoction

Drink eight ounces of the warm strained decoction (tea), once during the day as needed.

Dosage for Powder

This formula should be taken once daily. The powder can be used in several different ways. Make a smoothie, by adding twenty to thirty grams of the powder to eight ounces of juice smoothie, mix well, and drink. If that is an issue we recommend adding twenty to thirty grams of the powdered herbs to 00-size capsules. For more detailed instructions, follow the step-by-step guide for preparing a smoothie or capsules discussed in Chapter Five.

Herbal Ingredients

Grams	Chinese Herb	Botanical Name	Common Name
4.5	Bai Zhu 白朮	*Atractylodes*	Atractylodes
6	Cang Zhu 草烏	*Atractylodes* Lancea	Atractylodes
9	Dang Gui 當歸	*Angelica*	Angelica
9	Fang Feng 防風	*Ledebouriellae*	Siler
6	Ge Gen 葛根	*Puerariae*	Kudzu
9	Huang Qin 黃芩	*Schutellaria*	Baikal Skullcap
6	Ku Shen 苦參	*Sophora Flavescens*	Sophora
15	Qiang Huo 羌活	*Notopterygum*	Notopteygium
6	Ren Shen 人參	*Ginseng*	Ginseng
6	Sheng Ma 升麻	*Cimicifuga*	Cimicguga
15	Yin Chen 茵陈	*Artemisia*	Wormwood
9	Ze Xie 澤瀉	*Alisma Orientalis*	Water Plantain
15	Zhi Gan Cao 甘草	*Glycyrrhizae*	Licorice
9	Zhi Mu 知母	*Anemarrhena*	Anemarrhena
9	Zhu Ling 豬苓	*Polyporus*	Polyporus

Note
As with all STD it is advisable to treat all sexual partners to avoid reinfection.

Long Dan Xie Gan Tang
Gentiana Decoction to Drain the Liver

Therapeutic Actions
This prescription is used to treat gonorrhea; it relieves the symptoms of gonorrhea, syphilis, herpes zoster, and abnormal vaginal discharge.

Preparation

Traditionally, this formula was used in the raw form to prepare a decoction; however, for those who have not developed the taste for harsh teas, we suggest the user have the ingredients ground into a fine powder by his/her herb supplier, and then store the powder in a brown or amber glass bottle with a lid. Store it in a cool environment free of sunlight and moisture until needed — do not refrigerate.

Dosage for Tang or Decoction

Drink four ounces of the warm strained decoction (tea), three times during the day as needed.

Dosage for Powder

This formula should be taken twice daily. The powder can be used in several different ways. Make a smoothie, by adding twenty to thirty grams of the powder to eight ounces of juice smoothie, mix well, and drink. If that is an issue we recommend adding twenty to thirty grams of the powdered herbs to 00-size capsules. For more detailed instructions, follow the step-by-step guide for preparing a smoothie or capsules discussed in Chapter Five.

Herbal Ingredients

Grams	Chinese Herb	Botanical Name	Common Name
6	Chai Hu 柴胡	*Bupleurum*	Bupleurum
9	Che Qian Zi 車前子	*Plantago*	Plantago Seed
9	Chuan Mu Tong 川木通	*Clematis*	Clematis
3	Dang Gui 當歸	*Angelica*	Angelica
6	Gan Cao 甘草	*Glycyrrhiza*	Licorice
9	Huang Qin 黃芩	*Schutellaria*	Baikal Skullcap
6	Long Dan 龙胆	*Gentiana Scabra*	Gentian
9	Shu Di Huang 熟地黃	*Rehmanniae Preparata*	Rehmannia Cooked
12	Ze Xie 澤瀉	*Alisma Orientalis*	Water Plantain
9	Zhi Zi 梔子	*Gardenia*	Gardenia

Treatment Note

If there is excessive itching in the genital region, prepare a topical treatment by adding two additional herbs to the above decoction (tea) add nine grams each of the following two herbs to the above prescription: She Chuang Zi (fructus cnidii) and Ku Shen (radix sophorae flavescentis), and after cooking the tea for thirty minutes strain off all herbs and discard them, allow the tea to cool to room temperature and using a sterile cloth apply the liquid (tea) topically to the affected area for fifteen to thirty minutes. Repeat as necessary. You may use this tea several times before discarding it, to keep it fresh simply store it in the refrigerator. Do not drink this revised formula; it is a topical treatment!

Note

As with all STD it is advisable to treat all sexual partners to avoid reinfection.

❦

GOUT

Gout is a metabolic disorder that causes attacks of arthritis, usually in a single joint. It may be related to kidney stones and ultimately may lead to kidney failure. Most commonly, the joint affected is the joint at the base of the big toe, but it can affect other joints including the knee, ankle, wrist, foot, and small joints of the hand.

Symptoms include redness, swelling, tenderness, and pain. The redness and swelling may spread and be confused with cellulitis (inflammation of the connective tissue). The intensity of the pain and tenderness experienced by someone suffering from gout can be so severe that the person may not be able to stand on an affected foot or even tolerate the pressure of bedclothes on it.

Normally a diagnosis is confirmed by a blood test that shows high levels of uric acid. Increased levels of purine (a product of DNA) can increase uric acid levels therefore, even though a lot of Western physicians don't stress the importance of a strict low-purine diet, I believe people with gout should consider avoiding foods high in purine such as liver and other organ meats, legumes, poultry, and excess alcohol consumption. The last antagonist (alcohol) is known to trigger attacks of the disease and should be avoided or used with caution.

Along with the dietary suggestions, the following herbal prescriptions can be used to treat gout; also included are processing instructions and the formula's therapeutic action.

RAW HERB FORMULAS
Dang Gui Nian Tong Tang
Tangkuei Decoction to Lift the Pain

Therapeutic Actions
This formula is used to treat gout; it will heal the symptoms of arthritis and gout with swelling and inflammation, joint pain affecting the joints and extremities, with redness, swelling, and inflammation; heavy sensation in the shoulders and back; fullness in the chest and epigastrium.

Preparation
Traditionally, this formula was used in the raw form to prepare a decoction; however, for those who have not developed the taste for harsh teas, we suggest the user have the ingredients ground into a fine powder by his/her herb supplier, and then store the powder in a brown or amber glass bottle with a lid.

Store it in a cool environment free of sunlight and moisture until needed — do not refrigerate.

Dosage for Tang or Decoction
Drink eight ounces of the warm strained decoction (tea), once during the day as needed.

Dosage for Powder

This formula should be taken once daily. The powder can be used in several different ways. Make a smoothie, by adding twenty to thirty grams of the powder to eight ounces of juice smoothie, mix well, and drink. If that is an issue we recommend adding twenty to thirty grams of the powdered herbs to 00-size capsules. For more detailed instructions, follow the step-by-step guide for preparing a smoothie or capsules discussed in Chapter Five.

Herbal Ingredients

Grams	Chinese Herb	Botanical Name	Common Name
4.5	Bai Zhu 白朮	*Atractylodes*	Atractylodes
6	Cang Zhu 草烏	*Atractylodes Lancea*	Atractylodes
9	Dang Gui 當歸	*Angelica*	Angelica
9	Fang Feng 防風	*Ledebouriellae*	Siler
6	Ge Gen 葛根	*Puerariae*	Kudzu
9	Huang Qin 黃芩	*Schutellaria*	Baikal Skullcap
6	Ku Shen 苦參	*Sophora Flavescens*	Sophora
15	Qiang Huo 羌活	*Notopterygum*	Notopteygium
6	Ren Shen 人參	*Ginseng*	Ginseng
6	Sheng Ma 升麻	*Cimicifuga*	Cimicguga
15	Yin Chen 茵陈	*Artemisia*	Wormwood
9	Ze Xie 澤瀉	*Alisma Orientalis*	Water Plantain
15	Zhi Gan Cao 甘草	*Glycyrrhizae*	Licorice
9	Zhi Mu 知母	*Anemarrhena*	Anemarrhena
9	Zhu Ling 豬苓	*Polyporus*	Polyporus

Gui Zhi Shao Yao Zhi Mu Tang

Cinnamon Twig, Peony, and Anemarrhena Decoction

Therapeutic Actions

This formula is used to treat gout; it will heal the symptoms of arthritis, peri-arthritis of the shoulder, and gout with swelling and inflammation, joint pain affecting the joints and extremities, with redness, swelling, and inflammation; heavy sensation in the shoulders and back; swollen feet, dizziness, numbness of the extremities, and difficulty in walking and moving.

Preparation
Traditionally, this formula was used in the raw form to prepare a decoction; however, for those who have not developed the taste for harsh teas, we suggest the user have the ingredients ground into a fine powder by his/her herb supplier, and then store the powder in a brown or amber glass bottle with a lid. Store it in a cool environment free of sunlight and moisture until needed — do not refrigerate.

*Preparation Notes
The herb Sheng Jiang or fresh ginger should not be cooked for longer than five minutes. Do not add it to the herbs being cooked until the last five minutes of preparation time.

Dosage for Tang or Decoction
Drink eight ounces of the warm strained decoction (tea), once during the day as needed.

Dosage for Powder
This formula should be taken once daily. The powder can be taken in several different ways. Make a smoothie, by adding twenty to thirty grams of the powder to eight ounces of juice smoothie, mix well, and drink. If that is an issue we recommend adding twenty to thirty grams of the powdered herbs to 00-size capsules. For more detailed instructions, follow the step-by-step guide for preparing a smoothie or capsules discussed in Chapter Five.

Herbal Ingredients

Grams	Chinese Herb	Botanical Name	Common Name
6	Bai Qian 白前	*Cynanchum*	Cynanchum
9	Bai Shao 白芍	*Paeonia*	White Peony
15	Bai Zhu 白朮	*Atractylodes*	Atractylodes
12	Fang Feng 防風	*Ledebouriellae*	Siler
6	Fu Zi 附子	*Aconditum*	Aconite
6	Gan Cao 甘草	*Glycyrrhiza*	Licorice
12	Gui Zhi 桂枝	*Cinnamomum*	Cinnamon Twigs
15	Sheng Jiang* 生姜	*Zingiber Officinale*	Ginger, Sliced
12	Zhi Mu 知母	*Anemarrhena*	Anemarrhena

Juan Bi Tang

Remove Painful Obstruction Decoction

Therapeutic Actions

This formula is used to treat gout; it will heal the symptoms of osteoarthritis, rheumatoid arthritis, gout, bursitis, "frozen" shoulder, and pain and stiffness in the lower extremities. As well as joint pain that affects the joints and extremities, with redness, swelling, and inflammation; heavy sensation in the shoulders and back; fullness in the chest and epigastrium.

Preparation

Traditionally, this formula was used in the raw form to prepare a decoction; however, for those who have not developed the taste for harsh teas, we suggest the user have the ingredients ground into a fine powder by his/her herb supplier, and then store the powder in a brown or amber glass bottle with a lid. Store it in a cool environment free of sunlight and moisture until needed — do not refrigerate.

Dosage for Tang or Decoction

Drink eight ounces of the warm strained decoction (tea), once during the day as needed.

Dosage for Powder

This formula should be taken once daily. The powder can be used in several different ways. Make a smoothie, by adding twenty to thirty grams of the powder to eight ounces of juice smoothie, mix well, and drink. If that is an issue we recommend adding twenty to thirty grams of the powdered herbs to 00-size capsules. For more detailed instructions, follow the step-by-step guide for preparing a smoothie or capsules discussed in Chapter Five.

Herbal Ingredients

Grams	Chinese Herb	Botanical Name	Common Name
45	Chi Shao 赤芍	*Paeonia*	Red Peony
45	Dang Gui 當歸	*Angelica*	Angelica
45	Fang Feng 防風	*Ledebouriellae*	Siler
45	Huang Qin 黃芩	*Schutellaria*	Baikal Skullcap
45	Jiang Huang 姜黃	*Curcuma*	Turmeric
45	Qiang Huo 羌活	*Notopterygum*	Notopteygium
15	Zhi Gan Cao 甘草	*Glycyrrhizae*	Licorice

HANGOVER

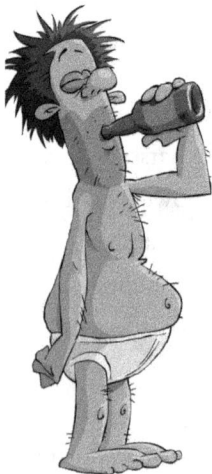

It's the morning after… and you awaken to the familiar side-effects from overindulging in alcohol, only to find yourself in bed with a complete stranger, naked, except for your shoes and socks, struggling to figure out how you got there and where in hell you parked your car.

Normally, two things determine the severity of a hangover; the amount and the type of alcohol consumed. Due to their high concentration of congeners (by-products of fermentation), generally speaking brandy, bourbon, and red wine produce the worst hangovers. Typical symptoms include: headache, nausea, stomachache, diarrhea, dehydration, vertigo, and bad breath.

One of the keys to a speedy recovery is replenishing body fluid by drinking large amounts of water. Sweating either through physical exercise, sauna or hot tub, can also help to relieve the side-effects of hangover—by purging the body of residual toxins from excessive amounts of alcohol. Fluid consumption (drinking lots of water) is critical when sweating or purging in order to replenish the fluid that is being excreted through perspiration.

Chinese herbal medicine can be very effective in treating the symptoms of a hangover, and will quickly restore sobriety. A point worth considering, when deciding the best way to use Chinese herbs to alleviate a hangover, is although patent formulas (herbal pills) are far more convenient, they do not replenish body fluid and re-hydrate the body like herbs that are decocted and consumed in tea form. An added benefit is that the body assimilates herbal tea faster than herbs in pill form.

Therefore even though patent formulas can be effective, decocting is the preferred method for preparing Chinese herbs when treating a hangover. And, the herbal tea should be drunk at room temperature (tepid), not hot.

The herbal prescriptions that follow can be effectively used to treat hangover and relieve the nausea, stomach ache, headache, diarrhea, de-hydration, vertigo and lack of energy. For each prescription, I will provide its unique processing instructions and therapeutic action.

RAW HERB FORMULA
Ge Hua Jie Cheng San
Pueraria Flower Powder for Detoxification and Awakening

Therapeutic Actions
This prescription is used to relieve the symptoms of a hangover; it will stop vomiting, relieve headache, dizziness, chest distention, lack of appetite and fatigue. Use for quick recovery from alcohol intoxication, this formula is famous for its ability to quickly restore sobriety.

Preparation

Traditionally, this formula was used in the raw form to prepare a decoction; however, for those who have not developed the taste for harsh teas, we suggest the user have the ingredients ground into a fine powder by his/her herb supplier, and then store the powder in a brown or amber glass bottle with a lid. Store it in a cool environment free of sunlight and moisture until needed — do not refrigerate.

Dosage for Tang or Decoction

Make a tea by adding nine grams of the powder to eight ounces of boiling water allow it to steep for fifteen minute and drink. Do this three times during the day or as needed.

Dosage for Powder

This formula should be taken twice daily. The powder can be used in several different ways. Make a smoothie, by adding twenty to thirty grams of the powder to eight ounces of juice smoothie, mix well, and drink. If that is an issue we recommend adding twenty to thirty grams of the powdered herbs to 00-size capsules. For more detailed instructions, follow the step-by-step guide for preparing a smoothie or capsules discussed in Chapter Five.

Herbal Ingredients

Grams	Chinese Herb	Botanical Name	Common Name
15	Bai Dou Kou 白豆蔻	*Amomim*	Cardamom
6	Bai Zhu 白朮	*Atractylodes*	Atractylodes
4.5	Chen Pi 陳皮	*Citrus Reticulate*	Tangerine Peel
4.5	Fu Ling 茯苓	*Poria Cocos*	Tuckahoe
6	Gan Jiang 乾薑	*Zingiber*	Ginger Dried
15	Ge Hua 葛花	*Flos Puerariae*	Kudzu
0.9	Lian Fang 蓮房	*Nelumbo*	Lotus Leaf
1.5	Mu Xiang 木香	*Aucklandiae*	Costus
1.5	Qing Pi 青皮	*Citrus Reticulata*	Tangerine Peel
4.5	Ren Shen 人參	*Ginseng*	Ginseng
15	Sha Ren 砂仁	*Amomum*	Amomum
6	Shen Qu 神曲	*Massa*	Leaven
6	Ze Xie 澤瀉	*Alisma Orientalis*	Water Plantain
4.5	Zhu Ling 豬苓	*Polyporus*	Polyporus

PATENT HERB FORMULAS
Bao Ji Wan
Po Chi Pills, Protect and Benefit Pills

Therapeutic Actions
This patent formula is used to treat the symptoms of a hangover or heartburn; including nausea, bloating, stomach cramping, vomiting, and diarrhea.

Caution
Do not use if pregnant.

Packaged
In box containing ten vials of pills.

Dosage
Take the full contents of one to two vials up to three times daily.

Kang Ning Wan
Pill Curing

Therapeutic Actions
This patent formula is used to treat the symptoms of a hangover; including belching, nausea, vomiting, and abdominal cramping.

Caution
Do not use during pregnancy.

Packaged
In box containing ten vials.

Dosage
Take the full contents of one to two vials up to three times daily.

HEARTBURN

Burning pain in the center of the chest that travels from the tip of the breastbone to the throat and on more than one occasion has been mistaken for a more serious heart condition, such as a heart attack.

Heartburn is usually a result of overeating rich or spicy foods, too much alcohol consumption, or a combination of the two.

Recurrent heartburn is a symptom of esophagitis, which is usually caused by acid reflux (the backflow of stomach acid) that often causes a burning sensation in the throat, is associated with the inability of the lower esophageal segment to close completely and in some cases is accompanied by a hiatal hernia.

Heartburn is often brought on either by lying down or bending forward, therefore you should avoid lying down flat and try lying with the upper body elevated, or sitting up.

Occasionally heartburn can cause chest pain so severe it has caused the sufferer to rush to a hospital emergency room believing that he/she was having a heart attack only to joyfully discover it was merely a severe case of indigestion.

Successful Chinese herbal treatment focuses on relieving heartburn, excessive belching, abdominal fullness, nausea, stomach cramping, vomiting, diarrhea and acid reflux. Once the herbs have addressed the underlying cause, full recovery is possible without permanent damage to the esophagus or digestive system.

All of the herbal prescriptions that follow can be effectively used to treat heartburn. For each prescription, I will provide its unique processing instructions and therapeutic action.

RAW HERB FORMULA
Xiang Sha Liu Jun Zi Tang
Six Gentlemen Decoction

Therapeutic Actions
This formula is used to treat the symptoms of heartburn, as well as gastritis, acid reflux and morning sickness, with excessive belching and abdominal fullness.

Preparation
Traditionally, this formula was used in the raw form to prepare a decoction; however, for those who have not developed the taste for harsh teas, we suggest the user have the ingredients ground into a fine powder by his/her herb supplier, and then store the powder in a brown or amber glass bottle with a lid. Store it in a cool environment free of sunlight and moisture until needed — do not refrigerate.

*Preparation Note
The herb Sheng Jiang or fresh ginger should not be cooked for longer than five minutes. Do not add it to the herbs being cooked until the last five minutes of preparation time.

Dosage for Tang or Decoction
Drink four to eight ounces of the warm strained decoction (tea), two to three times during the day as needed.

Dosage for Powder
This formula should be taken twice daily. The powder can be used in several different ways. Make a smoothie, by adding twenty to thirty grams of the powder to eight ounces of juice smoothie, mix well, and drink. If that is an issue we recommend adding twenty to thirty grams of the powdered herbs to 00-size capsules. For more detailed instructions, follow the step-by-step guide for preparing a smoothie or capsules discussed in Chapter Five.

Herbal Ingredients

Grams	Chinese Herb	Botanical Name	Common Name
6	Bai Zhu 白朮	*Atractylodes*	Atractylodes
3	Ban Xia 半夏	*Pinellia Ternata*	Half Summer
2.4	Chen Pi 陳皮	*Citrus Reticulate*	Tangerine Peel
6	Fu Ling 茯苓	*Poria Cocos*	Tuckahoe
2.1	Gan Cao 甘草	*Glycyrrhiza*	Licorice
2.1	Mu Xiang 木香	*Aucklandiae Lappa*	Costus
3	Ren Shen 人参	*Ginseng*	Ginseng
2.4	Sha Ren 砂仁	*Amomum*	Amomum Fruit
6	Sheng Jiang* 生姜	*Zingiber Officinale*	Ginger Sliced

PATENT HERB FORMULA

Bao Ji Wan

Po Chi Pills, Protect & Benefit Pills

Therapeutic Actions

This patent formula is used to treat the symptoms of a hangover or heartburn; including nausea, bloating, stomach cramping, vomiting, and diarrhea.

Caution

Do not use if pregnant.

Packaged

In box containing ten vials of pills.

Dosage

Take the full contents of one to two vials up to three times daily.

🍁

HEPATITIS B AND C

Hepatitis is an inflammation of the liver that can be either acute (of limited duration) or chronic (continuing). Acute hepatitis, the most common form, is usually caused by infection from a virus (as in viral hepatitis type B, which I will discuss below), a drug overdose, or exposure to certain chemicals. Acute hepatitis can also affect heavy drinkers who suffer from progressive liver disease. The most obvious symptom is jaundice, often preceded by nausea, vomiting, loss of appetite, aching muscles and joints, and tenderness in the upper right side of the abdomen.

There are three forms of viral hepatitis: type A, B and C. The focus here will be on types B and C.

Hepatitis B is an infectious inflammatory illness of the liver caused by the hepatitis B virus (HBV) that affects hominoidea, including humans. Originally known as serum hepatitis, the disease has caused epidemics in parts of Asia and Africa, and is epidemic in China.

The hepatitis B virus is transmitted by exposure to infectious blood or body fluids such as semen and vaginal fluid, while viral DNA has been detected in the saliva, tears, and urine of chronic carriers. Other risk factors for developing HBV infection include working in a healthcare setting, transfusions, dialysis, acupuncture, tattooing, sharing razors or toothbrushes with an infected person, traveling in countries where it is epidemic and residence in an institution.

The acute illness causes inflammation of the liver, vomiting, jaundice and rarely death. Chronic hepatitis B may eventually cause cirrhosis, and liver cancer. Although the disease has a poor response to all but a few current therapies, the infection is preventable by vaccination.

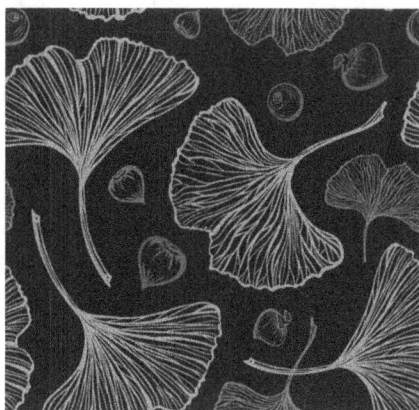

Hepatitis C is an infectious disease primarily affecting the liver, caused by the hepatitis C virus (HCV) which only infects humans and chimpanzees. The infection is often asymptomatic, but chronic infection can lead to scarring of the liver and ultimately to cirrhosis. In some cases, those with cirrhosis will go on to develop liver failure, liver cancer or life-threatening esophageal and gastric varices.

HCV is primarily spread by blood to blood contact associated with intravenous drug use, poorly sterilized medical equipment and transfusions.

Standard Western medical treatment involves the use of peginterferon and ribavirin, with either boceprevir or teleprivir added in some cases. Overall there is a fifty to eighty percent cure rate. Those who develop cirrhosis or liver cancer may require a transplant. Hepatitis C is the leading reason for liver transplantation. No vaccine against hepatitis is currently available.

In traditional Chinese medicine formulas containing fruit of the gardenia (Zhi Zi) and bupleurum hare's ear root (Chai Hu) are often the main ingredients in prescriptions used for treating hepatitis, as well as using antibiotic herbs that eliminate infection. Successful herbal treatment focuses on formulas that treat the jaundice, and relieve nausea, vomiting, loss of appetite, weakness, sore muscles and joints, and tenderness in the upper right side of the abdomen. Chinese herbs will address the underlying cause of hepatitis and treating the symptoms, but it is important for the user to discontinue using alcohol and/or drugs. If this is carried out, patients with hepatitis A or B should recover fully; however, at this time hepatitis C cannot be totally cured. The best traditional Chinese medicine can offer is an improved quality of life for those who suffer from hepatitis C.

All of the herbal prescriptions that follow can be effectively used to treat Hepatitis B and C. For each prescription, I will provide its unique processing instructions and therapeutic action.

RAW HERB FORMULAS
Da Chai Hu Tang
Major Bupleurum Decoction

Therapeutic Actions
This prescription is used to treat hepatitis; it relieves chills and fever, fullness of chest and the upper part of the abdomen, vomiting, depression, distension, and pain in the epigastrium (the upper central region of the abdomen), constipation or discharge of fluids rectally.

Preparation
Traditionally, this formula was used in the raw form to prepare a decoction; however, for those who have not developed the taste for harsh teas, we suggest the user have the ingredients ground into a fine powder by his/ her herb supplier, and then store the powder in a brown or amber glass bottle with a lid. Store it in a cool environment free of sunlight and moisture until needed — do not refrigerate.

*Preparation Note
The herb Sheng Jiang or fresh ginger should not be cooked for longer than five minutes. Do not add it to the herbs being cooked until the last five minutes of preparation time.

Dosage for Tang or Decoction
Drink eight ounces of the warm strained decoction (tea), three times during the day as needed.

Dosage for Powder
This formula should be taken two to three times daily. The powder can be used in several different ways. Make a smoothie, by adding twenty to thirty grams of the powder to eight ounces of juice smoothie, mix well, and drink. If that is an issue we recommend adding twenty to thirty grams of the powdered herbs to 00-size capsules. For more detailed instructions, follow the step-by-step guide for preparing a smoothie or capsules discussed in Chapter Five.

Herbal Ingredients

Grams	Chinese Herb	Botanical Name	Common Name
9	Bai Shao 白芍	*Paeonia*	White Peony
9	Ban Xia 半夏	*Pinellia Ternata*	Half Summer
24	Chai Hu 柴胡	*Bupleurum*	Bupleurum
6	Da Huang 大黄	*Rheum Palmatum*	Rhubarb Root
12 Pieces	Da Zao 大棗	*Ziziphus Jujuba*	Jujube
9	Huang Qin 黃芩	*Schutellaria*	Baikal Skullcap
15	Sheng Jiang* 生姜	*Zingiber Officinale*	Ginger, Sliced
4	Zhi Shi 炒枳實	*Citrus Aurantium*	Bitter Orange

Ren Shen Yang Ying Tang

Ginseng Decoction to Nourish the Nutritive Chi

Therapeutic Actions

This formula is used to treat hepatitis C; it treats the symptoms of fatigue, weakness, insomnia, shortness of breath, dizziness, dry throat and lips.

Preparation

Traditionally, this formula was used in the raw form to prepare a decoction; however, for those who have not developed the taste for harsh teas, we suggest the user have the ingredients ground into a fine powder by his/her herb supplier, and then store the powder in a brown or amber glass bottle with a lid. Store it in a cool environment free of sunlight and moisture until needed — do not refrigerate.

*Preparation Note

The herb Sheng Jiang or fresh ginger should not be cooked for longer than five minutes. Do not add it to the herbs being cooked until the last five minutes of preparation time.

Dosage for Tang or Decoction

Drink eight ounces of the warm strained decoction (tea), two to three times during the day as needed.

Dosage for Powder

This formula should be taken twice daily. The powder can be used in several different ways. Make a smoothie, by adding twenty to thirty grams of the powder to eight ounces of juice smoothie, mix well, and drink. If that is an issue we recommend adding twenty to thirty grams of the powdered herbs to 00-size capsules. For more detailed instructions, follow the step-by-step guide for preparing a smoothie or capsules discussed in Chapter Five.

Herbal Ingredients

Grams	Chinese Herb	Botanical Name	Common Name
18	Bai Shao 白芍	*Paeonia*	White Peony
6	Bai Zhu 白术	*Atractylodes*	Atractylodes
6	Chen Pi 陳皮	*Citrus Reticulate*	Tangerine Peel
9	Dang Gui 當歸	*Angelica*	Angelica
4	Fu Ling 茯苓	*Poria Cocos*	Tuckahoe
12	Huang Qi 黃芪	*Astragalus*	Milkvetch Root
6	Ren Shen 人參	*Ginseng*	Ginseng
3	Rou Gui 肉桂	*Cinnamomum*	Cinnamon Bark
3	Sheng Jiang* 生姜	*Zingiber Officinale*	Ginger Sliced
9	Shu Di Huang 熟地黃	*Rehmanniae Preparata*	Rehmannia Cooked
4	Wu Wei Zi 五味子	*Schisandra*	Schizandra
4	Yuan Zhi 遠志	*Polygala Tenuifolia*	Milkwort
3	Zhi Gan Cao 甘草	*Glycyrrhizae*	Licorice

PATENT HERB FORMULAS
Chuan Xin Lian – Antiphlogistic Pills

Andrographis Fight Inflammation Pills

Note

For the most effective treatment of hepatitis combine use with the patent formula Li Gan Pian.

Therapeutic Actions

This patent formula is used to treat hepatitis. It will also heal infections, skin abscesses, ulcers, and sores.

Cautions

Limit use to one week as prolonged use may lead to epigastric pain and diminished digestive function. Do not use if pregnant.

Packaged

In bottle of thirty six or one hundred coated pills, each 1.3 grams.

Dosage

Take two to three pills, three times per day. Dosage can be increased to five pills, every three hours, if needed.

Ji Gu Cao Wan

Abrus Pills

Note

For the most effective treatment of hepatitis combine use with Hsiao Yao Wan.

Therapeutic Actions

This patent formula is used to treat hepatitis; it relieves fever, fullness of chest and the upper part of the abdomen, vomiting, depression, distension and pain, constipation or diarrhea.

Packaged

In bottle of one hundred pills.

Dosage

Take four pills, three times per day. Dosage can be increased to eight pills, if needed.

Hsiao Yao Wan

Bupleurum Sedative Pills

Note: For the most effective treatment of hepatitis combine use with Ji Gu Cao Wan.

Therapeutic Actions

This patent formula is used to treat hepatitis; it relieves fever, fullness of chest and the upper part of the abdomen, vomiting, depression, distension and pain, constipation or diarrhea.

Caution

Do not use if you have PMS.

Packaged

In bottle of two hundred pills.

Dosage

Take eight pills, two to three times per day. Dosage can be increased to twelve pills, if needed.

Li Gan Pian

Benefit Liver Tablets

Note

For a more effective treatment of hepatitis combine use with the patent formula Chuan Xin Lian.

Therapeutic Actions

This patent formula is used to treat Infectious hepatitis and jaundice; it relieves chills and fever, fullness of chest and the upper part of the abdomen, vomiting, depression, distension and pain, constipation or diarrhea.

Caution

Do not take if you are suffering from cold or flu.

Packaged

In bottle of one hundred pills.

Dosage

Take four to six pills, three times per day.

❧

HERPES/GENITAL HERPES

Herpes is a sexually transmitted infection (STI), commonly referred to as a sexually transmitted disease (STD); a condition characterized by an eruption of small painful blisters on the skin. When a person is said to be suffering from herpes, it usually refers to an infection of the herpes simplex virus. Forms of the virus are responsible for cold sores (painful blisters around the lips) and for the sexually transmitted infection genital herpes, which is characterized by blisters on the sex organs. The virus can also cause a number of other conditions affecting the skin, mouth, eyes, brain, or in rare cases the entire body.

The herpes simplex virus should not be confused with two closely related viruses which are also characterized by skin blisters—the viracella-zoster virus, which is responsible for chickenpox, and herpes zoster, also known as shingles.

Genital herpes is a sexually transmitted disease that produces a painful rash on the genitals. Caused by the herpes simplex virus (Herpesvirus

Hominis, type 2) genital herpes is transmitted by sexual intercourse with an infected person.

After an incubation period of about a week, the virus produces itching, burning, soreness, and small blisters in the genital area. The blisters burst and leave small painful ulcers, which can last from ten to twenty-one days. The lymph nodes in the groin area may become enlarged and painful. The infected person may also feel sick, with headache and fever. Women with genital herpes may find that urination is painful if urine comes into contact with the sores. Occasionally there are cold sores around the mouth as well.

Once the virus enters the body it remains there for the rest of the person's life. Approximately forty-percent of those affected never have another attack after the first. Others however, suffer four or five attacks a year for several years. Gradually the attacks become less severe and the intervals between recurrences become longer.

The herpes virus may have a role in the development of cervical cancer. It is important for any woman who has herpes to have a cervical smear test (pap smear) every one to two years.

Successful Chinese medical treatment uses powerful herbal formulas that focus on treating the herpes virus, relieving the symptoms of infection including skin blisters, rash, itching, burning, sores, painful blisters and cold sores. Since full recovery is not possible as there is no known cure for herpes—an infected person should avoid spreading the virus by never engaging in unprotected sex when they are symptomatic.

As with all STD it is advisable to treat all sexual partners.

All of the herbal prescriptions that follow can be effectively used to treat herpes. For each prescription, I will provide its unique processing instructions and therapeutic action.

RAW HERB FORMULAS
Dao Chi San
Guide-out the Red Powder

Therapeutic Actions
This formula is used to treat genital herpes or oral herpes; characterized by symptoms of infection, stomatitis, and resolves sores, and dark-colored urine.

Preparation
Traditionally, this formula was used in the raw form to prepare a decoction; however, for those who have not developed the taste for harsh teas, we suggest the user have the ingredients ground into a fine powder by his/her herb supplier, and then store the powder in a brown or amber glass bottle with a lid. Store it in a cool environment free of sunlight and moisture until needed — do not refrigerate.

Dosage for Tang or Decoction
Drink four ounces of the warm strained decoction (tea), three times a day as needed.

Dosage for Powder
This formula should be taken twice daily. The powder can be used in several different ways. Make a smoothie, by adding twenty to thirty grams of the powder to eight ounces of juice smoothie, mix well, and drink. If that is an issue we recommend adding twenty to thirty grams of the powdered herbs to 00-size capsules. For more detailed instructions, follow the step-by-step guide for preparing a smoothie or capsules discussed in Chapter Five.

Herbal Ingredients

Grams	Chinese Herb	Botanical Name	Common Name
6	Chuan Mu Tong 川木通	*Clematis*	Clematis
6	Gan Cao 甘草	*Glycyrrhiza*	Licorice
6	Huang Lian 黃連	*Coptis*	Coptis
9	Mai Men Dong 麦冬	*Ophiopogon*	Winter Wheat
6	Shu Di Huang 熟地黃	*Rehmanniae Preparata*	Rehmannia Cooked
9	Zhu Ye 苦竹叶	*Phyllostachys*	Bamboo Leaves

Contraindication

Avoid heavily spiced food while taking this formula.

Note

As with all STD it is advisable to treat all sexual partners.

Long Dan Xie Gan Tang

Gentiana Decoction to Drain the Liver

Therapeutic Actions

This formula is used to treat genital herpes or oral herpes; characterized by symptoms of skin blisters, rash, itching, burning, sores, painful blisters and cold sores.

Preparation

Traditionally, this formula was used in the raw form to prepare a decoction; however, for those who have not developed the taste for harsh teas, we suggest the user have the ingredients ground into a fine powder by his/her herb supplier, and then store the powder in a brown or amber glass bottle with a lid. Store it in a cool environment free of sunlight and moisture until needed — do not refrigerate.

Dosage for Tang or Decoction

Drink four ounces of the warm strained decoction (tea), three times a day as needed.

Dosage for Powder

This formula should be taken twice daily. The powder can be taken in several different ways. Make a smoothie, by adding twenty to thirty grams of the powder to eight ounces of juice smoothie, mix well, and drink. If that is an issue we recommend adding twenty to thirty grams of the powdered herbs to 00-size capsules. For more detailed instructions, follow the step-by-step guide for preparing a smoothie or capsules discussed in Chapter Five.

Herbal Ingredients

Grams	Chinese Herb	Botanical Name	Common Name
6	Chai Hu 柴胡	*Bupleurum*	Bupleurum
9	Che Qian Zi 車前子	*Plantago*	Plantago Seed
9	Chuan Mu Tong 川木通	*Clematis*	Clematis
3	Dang Gui 當歸	*Angelica*	Angelica
6	Gan Cao 甘草	*Glycyrrhiza*	Licorice
9	Huang Qin 黄芩	*Schutellaria*	Baikal Skullcap
6	Long Dan 龙胆	*Gentiana Scabra*	Gentian
9	Shu Di Huang 熟地黄	*Rehmanniae Preparata*	Rehmannia Cooked
12	Ze Xie 澤瀉	*Alisma Orientalis*	Water Plantain
9	Zhi Zi 栀子	*Gardenia*	Gardenia

Contraindication

This formula should not be used for those with blood deficiencies.

Note

As with all STD it is advisable to treat all sexual partners.

🍁

HYPERTENSION

A person who has blood pressure resting blood pressure greater than 140mm Hg (systolic)/90mm Hg (diastolic) is clinically defined as having hypertension.

Hypertension usually causes no symptoms and generally goes undiscovered until detected by a physician during the course of a routine physical examination.

In ten percent of patients with elevated blood pressure, disorders of the kidneys, adrenal gland, and coarctation of the aorta, are the underlying cause of hypertension. However, the majority of people have no obvious cause; in such cases it is called essential hypertension.

It is well known that obesity, tobacco smoking, and heavy alcohol consumption, significantly increase the risk of hypertension. Smokers should stop smoking and heavy drinkers should drastically reduce their consumption of alcohol as well as restrict their intake of salt.

Possible complications of untreated high blood pressure include stroke, heart failure, kidney damage, and retinopathy (damage to the retina at the back of the eye). Severe hypertension may cause confusion and seizures.

Traditional Chinese herbal medicine can successfully treat hypertension using herbal formulas that focus on lowering blood pressure, improving circulation, and relieving chronic headaches, dizziness and increasing energy levels. However, reducing the amount of alcohol and/or drugs that are consumed and lowering his/her stress level is highly recommended.

All of the herbal prescriptions that follow can be effectively used to treat hypertension. For each prescription, I will provide its unique processing instructions and therapeutic action.

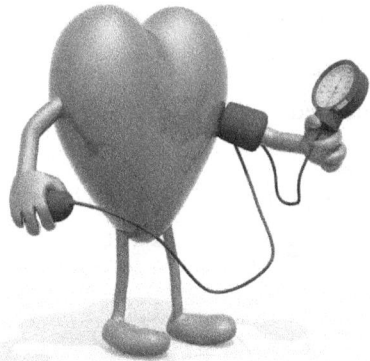

RAW HERB FORMULA
Wu Ling San
Five Ingredient Powder with Poria

Therapeutic Actions
This formula is used to treat hypertension and its symptoms, including but not limited to lack of energy, high blood pressure, poor circulation, dizziness, and headache, as well as treating cirrhosis, ascites and nephritis.

Preparation
Traditionally, this formula was used in the raw form to prepare a decoction; however, for those who have not developed the taste for harsh teas, we suggest the user have the ingredients ground into a fine powder by his/her herb supplier, and then store the powder in a brown or amber glass bottle with a lid.

Store it in a cool environment free of sunlight and moisture until needed — do not refrigerate.

Dosage for Tang or Decoction
Drink eight ounces of the warm strained decoction (tea), one–two times a day as needed.

Dosage for Powder
This formula should be taken twice daily. The powder can be taken in several different ways. Make a smoothie, by adding twenty to thirty grams of the powder to eight ounces of juice smoothie, mix well, and drink. If that is an issue we recommend adding twenty to thirty grams of the powdered herbs to 00-size capsules. For more detailed instructions, follow the step-by-step guide for preparing a smoothie or capsules discussed in Chapter Five.

Herbal Ingredients

Grams	Chinese Herb	Botanical Name	Common Name
9	Bai Zhu 白朮	*Atractylodes*	Atractylodes
9	Fu Ling 茯苓	*Poria Cocos*	Tuckahoe
6	Gui Zhi 桂枝	*Cinnamomum*	Cinnamon Twigs
15	Ze Xie 澤瀉	*Alisma Orientalis*	Water Plantain
9	Zhu Ling 豬苓	*Polyporus*	Polyporus

Contraindication

As this formula eliminates excess body fluids (through urination) it should not be used for a prolonged period of time by individuals who sweat profusely.

PATENT HERB FORMULA
Yu Feng Ning Xin Pian

Cure Wind and Calm the Heart Pill

Therapeutic Actions

This patent formula treats hypertension, dispels heat, generates fluids, stops thirst, relieves headache and dizziness, and alleviates diarrhea. It has been recently researched for its effects on <u>reducing cravings for alcohol</u>.

Packaged

In box of thirty tablets.

Dosage

Take five tablets three times daily. Note: In severe cases or during the early stages of treatment (the first two weeks) a fifty percent increase in dosage can be used, and reduced as the treatment takes effect.

🍁

INFECTION/SKIN ABSCESS, ULCERS AND SORES

Intravenous drug users are at increased risk for developing abscesses and other bacterial skin infections. Bacterial infections are usually caused by the users own communal bacteria. In other words, the bacteria naturally living on a healthy person's skin is usually the cause of a painful sometimes life-threatening infection.

When a needle comes in contact with dirt and bacteria on the skin, they are transferred into the epidermis, sometimes causing an infection. Consistent use of clean needles and rubbing alcohol before injection can reduce this risk but will not eliminate it entirely.

A bacterial skin abscess is one of the most common bacterial infections present among intravenous drug users. Although these infections will sometimes resolve on their own, left untreated they can lead to sepsis, amputation and even death.

Abscesses are usually round or oval shaped with dark pus-filled masses at the center. An abscess can develop anywhere on the body, but usually appear at or near the injection site. The result is pain, swelling, and tenderness to the touch. If it is allowed to grow unchecked, the abscess may spread into the bloodstream or into deeper tissue where it can create more serious health complications.

Traditional Chinese herbal medicine can successfully treat infection/skin abscesses, ulcers and sores using herbal formulas that focus on reducing the infection, draining pus, eliminating toxins, draining abscesses and other bacterial skin infections.

All of the herbal prescriptions that follow can be effectively used to treat infections/skin abscesses, ulcers and sores. For each prescription, I will provide its unique processing instructions and therapeutic action.

RAW HERB FORMULAS
Pai Nong San
Drain the Pus Powder

Therapeutic Actions
This prescription is used to treat infection, skin abscess, ulcers and sores; it relieves the symptoms of infection. It drains pus, eliminates toxins and drains abscess and nodules.

Preparation
Traditionally, this formula was used in the raw form to prepare a decoction; however, for those who have not developed the taste for harsh teas, we suggest the user have the ingredients ground into a fine powder by his/her herb supplier, and then store the powder in a brown or amber glass bottle with a lid. Store it in a cool environment free of sunlight and moisture until needed — do not refrigerate.

Dosage for Tang or Decoction
Drink eight ounces of the warm strained decoction (tea), one to two times a day as needed.

Dosage for Powder
This formula should be taken twice daily. The powder can be taken in several different ways. Make a smoothie, by adding twenty to thirty grams of the powder to eight ounces of juice smoothie, mix well, and drink. If that is an issue we recommend adding twenty to thirty grams of the powdered herbs to 00-size capsules. For more detailed instructions, follow the step-by-step guide for preparing a smoothie or capsules discussed in Chapter Five.

Herbal Ingredients

Grams	Chinese Herb	Botanical Name	Common Name
4.5	Bai Shao 白芍	*Paeonia*	White Peony
1.5	Jie Geng 桔梗	*Platycodon*	Platycodon
16 Pieces	Zhi Shi 炒枳實	*Citrus Aurantium*	Bitter Orange

Wu Wei Xiao Du Yin

Five-Ingredient Decoction to Eliminate Toxins

Therapeutic Actions

This prescription is used to treat infection, skin abscess, ulcers and sores; it relieves the infection and eliminates toxins from the body. It will dry-up external abscesses, ulcers and sores.

Preparation

Traditionally, this formula was used in the raw form to prepare a decoction; however, for those who have not developed the taste for harsh teas, we suggest the user have the ingredients ground into a fine powder by his/her herb supplier, and then store the powder in a brown or amber glass bottle with a lid. Store it in a cool environment free of sunlight and moisture until needed — do not refrigerate.

Dosage for Tang or Decoction (for internal use)

Drink eight ounces of the warm strained decoction (tea), one-two times a day as needed.

Dosage for Powder (for internal use)

This formula should be taken twice daily. The powder can be taken in several different ways. Make a smoothie, by adding twenty to thirty grams of the powder to eight ounces of juice smoothie, mix well, and drink. If that is an issue we recommend adding twenty to thirty grams of the powdered herbs to 00-size capsules. For more detailed instructions, follow the step-by-step guide for preparing a smoothie or capsules discussed in Chapter Five.

Treatment Note (for external use)

This prescription can be used "internally" (as described above) or it can be applied to the skin for "external" relief. To make an external wrap prepare a compress. An herbal compress is made by first decocting the herbs. After the tea is made, the herbs can either be strained and discarded, or left in the pot and allowed to cool. Leaving the herbs in the pot, increases the potency of the herbal mixture. Once prepared, the decocted tea can be re-used for approximately five to seven days by simply keeping the pot covered and re-heating when needed. It is not necessary to boil the herbal brew a second time as long as you keep the pot covered and reheat the decoction every day; it should not become rancid. However, if you are concerned about maintaining the freshness of the herbal tea, then I suggest you store it in a closed glass jar in the refrigerator and reheat – usable for up to two weeks when refrigerated. The compress is prepared by soaking sterile surgical gauze, or some other sterile soft cotton material, in the warm herbal tea, then the excess fluid is wrung out, and the cotton material is applied to the injured area. When making a compress, the cotton material should be saturated with the fluid, but not dripping. Then wrap the area with a warm towel or blanket to promote sweating. Repeat the process as necessary.

Herbal Ingredients

Grams	Chinese Herb	Botanical Name	Common Name
9	Jin Yin Hua 金银花	*Lonicera Japonica*	Honeysuckle
3-6	Pu Gong Ying 蒲公英	*Taraxacum*	Dandelion
3-6	Tian Kui Zi 天葵子	*Semiaquilegia*	Semiaquileqia
3-6	Ye Ju Hua 野菊花	*Chrysanthemum*	Chrysanthemum
3-6	Zi Hua Di Ding 紫花地丁	*Viola Yedoensis*	Tokyo Violet

Contraindication

Use with caution if you have digestive weakness.

PATENT HERB FORMULAS
Chuan Xin Lian – Antiphlogistic Pills
Andrographis Fight Inflammation Pills

Therapeutic Actions
This patent formula is used to treat infection, skin abscess, ulcers and sores; it will heal skin abscesses, ulcers, and sores.

Cautions
Prolonged use may lead to epigastric pain and diminished digestive function. Do not use if pregnant.

Packaged
In bottle of thirty six or one hundred coated pills, each 1.3 grams.

Dosage
Take two to three pills, three times per day. Dosage can be increase to five pills, every three hours, if needed.

Chuan Xin Lian Cream
Andrographis Anti-Inflammatory Ointment

Therapeutic Actions
This prescription is used to treat infection, skin abscess, ulcers and sores; it relieves infection in the skin, used for inflammatory skin disorders with redness, swelling and pain. Used topically on abscesses, boils, carbuncles and furuncles, acne, eczema, dermatitis and other inflamed skin conditions.

Caution
For external use only, avoid contact with the eyes or broken skin.

Packaged
In tube containing twenty grams of ointment.

Dosage
Apply locally to the affected area, three to four times per day.

Huang Lian Jie Du Wan
Coptis Resolve Toxin Pills

Therapeutic Actions
This patent formula is used to treat infection, skin abscess, ulcers and sores; it will heal skin abscesses, ulcers, and sores.

Cautions
Discontinue use if loose stools or epigastric pain becomes uncomfortable. This formula should not be used long-term.

Packaged
In bottle of two hundred pills.

Dosage
Take eight pills, three times per day. Dosage can be increased to twelve pills, if needed.

🍁

INFERTILITY

Infertility is the inability of a couple to conceive. Abuse of substances such as marijuana, alcohol, drugs etc. can all be contributing factors or a direct cause of infertility.

Conception depends on the production of healthy sperm by the man, healthy eggs by the woman, and sexual intercourse so the sperm reaches the woman's fallopian tubes.

There must not be any form of obstruction to prevent the sperm from reaching the egg, and the sperm must be able to fertilize the egg when they meet. The fertilized egg must be able to become implanted in the woman's uterus, the embryo must be healthy and its hormonal environment must be adequate for further development so that the pregnancy can continue to full term. Infertility may result from a disturbance of one or more of these factors.

Infertility usually increases with age; the older a couple is when trying to conceive, the more difficult it may be.

Traditional Chinese herbal medicine can successfully treat infertility using herbal formulas that focus on promoting healthy functioning of the reproductive system, for both men and women; they address lack of energy, and heal diseases that are known to affect fertility (such as: leukorrhea, irregular or painful menstruation, impotence, excessive seminal emissions, and frequent urination). Chinese medicine will balance progesterone levels, correct loss of libido and improve sperm mobility. Best results are achieved when the user stops or reduces their amount of alcohol/drugs use.

All of the herbal prescriptions that follow can be effectively used to treat infertility. For each prescription, I will provide its unique processing instructions and therapeutic action.

RAW HERB FORMULAS
Ai Fu Nuan Gong Wan
Mugwort and Cyperus Pill for Warming the Womb (for women only)

Therapeutic Actions
This prescription is used to treat infertility in women; it relieves deficiency and cold uterus; leukorrhea, sallow and yellowish facial complexion, painful limbs, lethargy, low energy, lack of appetite, irregular menstruation, and occasional lower abdominal pain.

Preparation
Traditionally, this formula was used in the raw form to prepare a decoction; however, for those who have not developed the taste for harsh teas, we suggest the user have the ingredients ground into a fine powder by his/

her herb supplier, and then store the powder in a brown or amber glass bottle with a lid. Store it in a cool environment free of sunlight and moisture until needed — do not refrigerate.

Dosage for Tang or Decoction

Drink four ounces of the warm strained decoction (tea), two to three times a day as needed.

Dosage for Powder

This formula should be taken twice daily. The powder can be taken in several different ways. Make a smoothie, by adding twenty to thirty grams of the powder to eight ounces of juice smoothie, mix well, and drink. If that is an issue we recommend adding twenty to thirty grams of the powdered herbs to 00-size capsules. For more detailed instructions, follow the step-by-step guide for preparing a smoothie or capsules discussed in Chapter Five.

Herbal Ingredients

Grams	Chinese Herb	Botanical Name	Common Name
6	Ai Ye 艾葉	*Artemisia Argyi*	Wormwood Leaf
6	Bai Shao 白芍	*Paeonia*	White Peony
6	Chuan Xiong 川芎	*Ligusticum*	Cnidium
6	Dang Gui 當歸	*Angelica*	Angelica
6	Huang Qi 黃芪	*Astragalus*	Milkvetch
3	Pu Huang 蒲黃炭	*Typha Angustifolia*	Bulrush
5	Rou Gui 肉桂	*Cinnamomum*	Cinnamon Bark
6	Shu Di Huang 熟地黃	*Rehmanniae Preparata*	Rehmannia Cooked
9	Tu Si Zi 菟絲子	*Cuscuta*	Dodder Seed
6	Wu Zhu Yu 吳茱萸	*Evodia Rutaecarpa*	Evodia
12	Xiang Fu 香附	*Cyperus*	Nutgrass
5	Xu Duan 續斷	*Dipsacus Asper*	Teasel
6	Yi Mu Cao 益母草	*Leonurus*	Motherwort

Contraindication

Avoid raw or cold foods during treatment.

You Gui Wan

Restore the Right Pills (for males only)

Therapeutic Actions

This prescription is used to treat infertility in males; it relieves infertility, impotence, seminal emissions and frequent urination.

Preparation

First powder the herbs and then prepare pills. For more information on preparing a pills read the step-by-step processing instructions discussed in Chapter Five.

*Dosage Note

The gram weight to be used in this formula is listed with a minimum/maximum range. This prescription should be prepared by using the lower dosage and only increase dosage to achieve stronger results when needed.

Dosage

Take fifteen grams of pills in the a.m. and again in the p.m.; do this daily for a minimum of three months.

Contraindications

Avoid cold and raw foods while taking this formula; refrain from consuming alcohol while taking this formula.

Herbal Ingredients

Grams	Chinese Herb	Botanical Name	Common Name
90	Dang Gui 當歸	*Angelica*	Angelica
120	Du Zhong 杜仲	*Eucommia*	Eucommia
60-180*	Fu Zi 附子	*Aconditum*	Aconite
120	Gou Qi Zi 枸杞子	*Lycii Fructus*	Wolfberry
120	Lu Jiao Jiao 鹿角胶	*Cervus Nippon*	Horn Gelatin
20	Rou Cong Rong 肉蓯蓉	*Cistanche*	Cistanche
60-120*	Rou Gui 肉桂	*Cinnamomum*	Cinnamon
120	Shan Yao 山药	*Dioscorea*	Yam
90	Shan Zhu Yu 山茱萸	*Corni Fructus*	Dogwood Fruit
240	Shu Di Huang 熟地黄	*Rehmanniae Preparata*	Rehmannia Cooked
120	Tu Si Zi 菟絲子	*Cuscuta*	Dodder Seed

PATENT HERB FORMULAS
Cu Yun Yu Tai Capsule
Aka Fu Nu Bao
Promote Pregnancy Pills (for women only)

Therapeutic Actions
This patent formula is used to treat infertility in females; it relieves the symptoms of primary and secondary infertility, irregular menstruation, long menstrual cycle, low or short progesterone phase of the menstrual cycle, weakness in the lower back, knees and legs, loss of libido, and general debility.

Cautions
Discontinue use during colds and flu, pregnancy, or for patients on anticoagulant therapy. Watch for bruising or an increased tendency to bleeding.

Packaged

In bottle of thirty six pills.

Dosage

Take three to four pills, three times per day.

Wu Zi Yan Zong Wan

Five-Seed Abundant Ancestors Pills (for men only)

Therapeutic Actions

This patent formula is used to treat infertility in males; it relieves the symptoms of kidney deficiency causing sexual dysfunction, impotence, premature ejaculation, infertility, lumbar pain and depression. This formula is effective at raising sperm count and increasing sperm motility.

Caution

Discontinue use during colds and flu.

Packaged

In bottle of two hundred pills.

Dosage

Take eight pills three times a day. Dosage can be increased to twelve pills, if needed.

Note

For the best results from this treatment, it is advised to minimize intercourse for a one to three month period while building up reserves (of sexual energy) while using this formula. After the end of the rebuilding phase, continue to take eight pills three times a day. Dosage can be increased to twelve pills, if needed.

❧

INSOMNIA

Insomnia is a fairly common problem in the U.S.; a national survey has shown that one in every three adults has trouble sleeping and that hypnotic drugs (sleeping pills) are among the most widely used of all prescription medicines.

Most insomnia sufferers complain of increased daytime fatigue, irritability, and difficulty coping. The most common cause of insomnia is worrying about problems, but other causes are implicated in about half of all cases.

Other causes include physical disorders such as sleep apnea, restless legs, environmental factors (such as noise and light), lifestyle factors (like excessive consumption of caffeine), and the misuse of anti-anxiety drugs (barbiturate drugs).

Insomnia can also be a symptom of psychiatric illness. People with anxiety and/or depression may have difficulty getting to sleep. Schizophrenia often causes people to pace at night, aroused by voices or delusions.

Most importantly, I should mention that withdrawal syndrome from hypnotic drugs, anti-depressants, tranquilizers, and narcotics, such as heroin may cause insomnia that can last for weeks.

Putting your body on a regular schedule (ending erratic hours), and increasing the amount of daily exercise, can both be helpful to cure insomnia along with the aid of Chinese herbal formulas. The successful use of Chinese herbs will help to calm the mind, as well as treat the insomnia, relieve the anxiety, and nervousness. I would also suggest that the user discontinue drug use until normal sleep patterns are developed.

All of the herbal prescriptions that follow can be effectively used to treat insomnia. For each prescription, I will provide its unique usage instructions and therapeutic action.

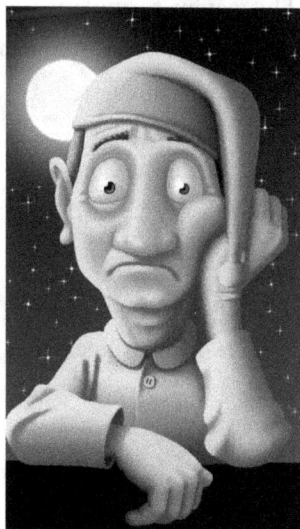

PATENT HERB FORMULAS
Shen Classic Tea
Calm Shen Nourish Heart Tea

Therapeutic Actions
This patent formula is used to treat insomnia; it relieves anxiety and nervousness due to stress, and disturbed Shen (in TCM this is a mental/ spiritual imbalance) causing insomnia, restlessness, and anxiety.

Packaged
In box of thirty tea bags.

Dosage
Drink one cup of hot tea, three times per day.

Suan Zao Ren Tang Pian
Zizyphus Decoction Tablet

Therapeutic Actions
This patent formula is used to treat insomnia; it relieves disturbed Shen causing insomnia, restlessness, anxiety, and has a sedative effect on the central nervous system.

Packaged
In bottle of forty eight pills.

Dosage
Take two pills, three times per day. Dosage can be increase to five pills, if needed.

JAUNDICE

Jaundice is the yellowing of the skin and the whites of the eyes that is caused by an accumulation of the bile pigment (bilirubin). Bilirubin is a brownish yellow substance found in bile. It is produced when the liver breaks down old red blood cells and is a symptom of many liver and biliary disorders such as cirrhosis, hepatitis, and liver disease, etc.

There are three types—hemolytic, hepatocellular, and obstructive. In hemolytic jaundice more bilirubin is produced than the liver is able to process. In hepatocellular jaundice, bilirubin builds up in the blood because its transfer from liver cells to bile is prevented, usually as the result of acute hepatitis or liver failure.

In obstructive jaundice, bile is prevented from flowing out of the liver because of disorders that cause a blockage of the bile ducts—such as gallstones or a tumor. Obstructive jaundice can also occur when the bile ducts have been destroyed as a result of biliary cirrhosis. Two other characteristic features that accompany obstructive jaundice are pale feces and dark urine.

The diagnostic procedures that are performed to determine the specific type of jaundice include blood smear, blood test, liver biopsy, ultrasound scanning, and liver function tests.

Jaundice is commonly found as a complication of liver diseases connected to excessive long-term alcohol and drug use. Successful Chinese medical treatment depends on the use of herbal formulas that focus on treating infectious hepatitis; reducing fever, invigorating liver functioning improves appetite, increases energy levels, and will slowly return skin and eye tone back to their natural color. It is imperative that the user discontinue their use of alcohol and drugs to avoid permanent irreparable damage to the organ.

All of the herbal prescriptions that follow can be effectively used to treat jaundice. For each prescription, I will provide its unique processing instructions and therapeutic action.

RAW HERB FORMULA
Yin Chen Hao Tang
Artemesia Scoparia Decoction

Therapeutic Actions
This formula treats infectious hepatitis and jaundice, and benefits the liver and gallbladder, reduces fever, invigorates the blood and relieves constipation by opening the bowels.

Preparation
Traditionally, this formula was used in the raw form to prepare a decoction; however, for those who have not developed the taste for harsh teas, we suggest the user have the ingredients ground into a fine powder by his/her herb supplier, and then store the powder in a brown or amber glass bottle with a lid. Store it in a cool environment free of sunlight and moisture until needed — do not refrigerate.

Dosage for Tang or Decoction
Drink four to eight ounces of the warm strained decoction (tea), one-two times a day as needed.

Dosage for Powder
This formula should be taken once or twice daily. The powder can be used in several different ways. Make a smoothie, by adding twenty to thirty grams of the powder to eight ounces of juice smoothie, mix well, and drink. If that is an issue we recommend adding twenty to thirty grams of the powdered herbs to 00-size capsules. For more detailed instructions, follow the step-by-step guide for preparing a smoothie or capsules discussed in Chapter Five.

Herbal Ingredients

Grams	Chinese Herb	Botanical Name	Common Name
6	Da Huang 大黃	*Rheum*	Rhubarb
18	Yin Chen 茵陈	*Artemisia*	Wormwood
9	Zhi Zi 栀子	*Gardenia*	Gardenia

Contraindication

This formula should not be used by pregnant women.

PATENT HERB FORMULAS
Ji Gu Cao Chong Ji
Arbus Instant Crystal Medicine

Therapeutic Actions

This patent formula is used to treats infectious hepatitis and jaundice; it is very useful for acute and chronic hepatitis.

Packaged

In box of ten packets, each contains twenty grams of instant crystal medicine.

Dosage

Take one packet mix with four to eight ounces of boiling water; drink three times daily.

Long Dan Xie Gan Wan
Gentiana Drain Liver Pills

Therapeutic Actions

This patent formula is used to treat hepatitis and jaundice.

Packaged

In bottle of two hundred pills.

Dosage

Take eight pills two to three times daily.

❧

LIVER CANCER

Liver cancer can present itself as a malignant tumor in the liver that may be primary cancer (originating in the liver itself) or secondary cancer (spread from elsewhere in the body). There are two main types of primary liver tumors a hepatoma, which develops in the liver cells, and a cholangiocarcinoma which comes from cells lining the bile duct.

Hepatomas are the most common form of liver cancer worldwide. They are closely linked to hepatitis B which is common throughout Africa, the Middle East, and the Far East.

In the U.S., hepatitis B is relatively uncommon so hepatomas are rarer. There are only about three or four new cases per one hundred thousand people annually. When a hepatoma does occur, it is usually a complication of cirrhosis of the liver caused by alcohol abuse.

The most common symptoms of liver cancer are weight loss, loss of appetite and lethargy. Additionally, there is also often pain in the upper right abdomen. Advanced stages of the disease are marked by jaundice and ascites (fluid retention in the abdomen). Liver tumors are usually detected as a result of ultrasound scanning that reveals abnormal areas in the liver. The diagnosis is confirmed by liver biopsy.

In cases where cirrhosis is not also present—which is rare in the U.S.—complete removal of the tumor leading to cure is sometimes possible. In other cases anticancer drugs are used in an attempt to prolong the life of the patient. Unfortunately there is no known cure for secondary liver cancer.

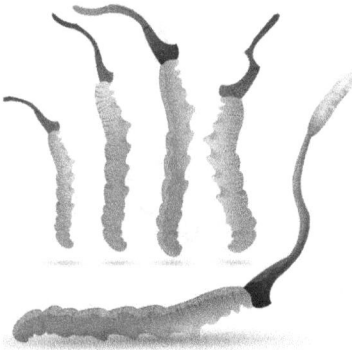

Chinese herbal medicine can be used to treat liver cancer; herbal formulas focus on treating the liver cirrhosis as well as liver cancer by softening hard masses. Chinese herbs can also be used to reduce distention (swelling), relieve pain, increase appetite, and return energy levels to normal. It is extremely important that the user stop using alcohol and drugs to achieve the best results.

All of the herbal prescriptions that follow can be effectively used to treat liver cancer. For each prescription, I will provide its unique processing instructions and therapeutic action.

A Word of Caution

No treatment of cancer is recommended without competent Western medical evaluation and guidance.

RAW HERB FORMULAS
Bie Jia Jian Wan
Soft-Shelled Turtle Shell Pill

Therapeutic Actions

This prescription is used to treat liver cirrhosis and liver cancer; it increases circulation of blood and Chi, relieves the body of dampness and dissolves phlegm, it softens hard masses, reduces distention and abdominal pain, and stops muscle wasting while improving the appetite.

Preparation

Traditionally, this formula is used in the raw form to prepare pills or capsules; the user should have the ingredients ground into a fine powder by his/her herb supplier, and then store the powder in a brown or amber glass bottle with a lid. Store it in a cool environment free of sunlight and moisture until needed — do not refrigerate.

Dosage for Using the Powder

This formula should be taken three times daily. The powder can be used in several different ways. Make a smoothie, by adding twenty to thirty grams of the powder to eight ounces of juice smoothie, mix well, and drink. If that is an issue we recommend adding twenty to thirty grams of the powdered herbs to 00-size capsules. For more detailed instructions, follow the step-by-step guide for preparing a smoothie or capsules discussed in Chapter Five.

Herbal Ingredients

Grams	Chinese Herb	Botanical Name	Common Name
37	Bai Shao 白芍	*Paeonia Lactiflora*	White Peony
7.5	Ban Xia 半夏	*Pinellia Ternata*	Half Summer
90	Bie Jia 鳖甲	*Trionyx Sinensis*	Turtle Shell
45	Chai Hu 柴胡	*Bupleurum*	Bupleurum
22.5	Da Huang 大黃	*Rheum Palmatum*	Rhubarb
22.5	E Jiao 阿胶	*Equus Asinus*	Ass-Hide Glue
30	Lu Feng Fang 露蜂	*Nidus Vespae*	Hornet's Nest
22.5	Gan Jiang 乾薑	*Zingiber Officinale*	Ginger Dried
22.5	Gui Zhi 桂枝	*Cinnamomum*	Cinnamon
22.5	Hou Po 厚朴	*Magnolia Officinalis*	Magnolia Bark
22.5	Huang Qin 黃芩	*Schutellaria*	Skullcap
22.5	Ling Xiao Hua 凌霄花	*Flos Campsis*	Trumpet Creeper
90	Mang Xiao 芒硝	*Natrii Sulfas*	Sodium Sulfate
37	Mu Dan Pi 牡丹皮	*Paeonia Suffruticosa*	Tree Peony
45	Qiang Lang 蜣螂	*Catharsium*	Dung Beetle
22.5	Qu Mai 瞿麦	*Dianthus Superbus*	Dianthus
7.5	Ren Shen 人参	*Panax Ginseng*	Ginseng
22.5	She Gan 射干	*Belamcanda*	Blackberry Lily
22.5	Shi Wei 石韦	*Pyrosia Sheareri*	Japanese Fern
22.5	Shu Fu Chong 鼠妇虫	*Armadillidium*	Pillbug
15	Tao Ren 桃仁	*Prunus Persica*	Peach Seed
7.5	Ting Li Zi 葶苈子	*Descurainia Sophia*	Lepidum
37	Tu Bei Chong 土鳖虫	*Eupolyphaga Sinensis*	Eupolyphaga

Treatment Note

TCM's use of this formula is typically for a minimum of six months; studies indicate longer use generated a more effective treatment.

Caution

Self-treating cancer is not recommended without competent Western medical evaluation and guidance.

Da Huang Zhe Chong Wan

Rhubarb and Eupolyphaga Pill

Therapeutic Actions

This prescription is used to treat liver cancer; it relieves chronic hepatitis, liver fibrosis, liver cirrhosis, liver cancer, and the symptoms of emaciation, abdominal distension with an inability to eat, dry mouth, rough and scaly skin, and dark appearance of the eyes with no spirit.

Preparation

Traditionally, this formula is used in the raw form to prepare pills or capsules; the user should have the ingredients ground into a fine powder by his/her herb supplier, and then store the powder in a brown or amber glass bottle with a lid. Store it in a cool environment free of sunlight and moisture until needed — do not refrigerate.

Dosage for Using the Powder

This formula should be taken twice daily. The powder can be taken in several different ways. Make a smoothie, by adding twenty to thirty grams of the powder to eight ounces of juice smoothie, mix well, and drink. If that is an issue we recommend adding twenty to thirty grams of the powdered herbs to 00-size capsules. For more detailed instructions, follow the step-by-step guide for preparing a smoothie or capsules discussed in Chapter Five.

Herbal Ingredients

Grams	Chinese Herb	Botanical Name	Common Name
120	Bai Shao 白芍	*Paeonia Lactiflora*	White Peony
300	Da Huang 大黃	*Rheum Palmatum*	Rhubarb
90	Gan Cao 甘草	*Glycyrrhiza*	Licorice
30	Gan Qi 幹漆	*Toxiodendron*	Dried Lacquer
60	Huang Qin 黃芩	*Schutellaria*	Baikal Skullcap
60	Ku Xing Ren 杏仁	*Prunus*	Apricot Seed
60	Meng Chong 虻蟲	*Tabanus Bivttatus*	Gadfly
60	Qi Cao 蛴螬	*Holotrichia Diamphala*	Coleopteran Larva
300	Shu Di Huang 地黃熟	*Rehmanniae Preparata*	Rehmannia Cooked
60	Shui Zhi 水蛭	*Hirudo Nipponica*	Leech, Dried
60	Tao Ren 桃仁	*Prunus Persica*	Peach Seed
30	Tu Bei Chong 土鱉虫	*Eupolyphaga*	Eupolyphaga

Contraindications

Use of this formula may be associated with mild diarrhea; however, this side-effect is self-limiting and does not require discontinuation of this formula. Another side-effect can be bleeding from the gums and nose – if that occurs temporarily discontinue use of the formula, then try taking it again. If bleeding persists or becomes profuse discontinue use entirely.

Treatment Note

TCM's use of this formula is typically for a minimum of six months; studies indicate longer use generated a more effective treatment.

Caution

Self-treating cancer is not recommended without competent Western medical evaluation and guidance.

PATENT HERB FORMULA
Zhi Yan Pian

Decancerlin Tablets aka Treat Cancer Tablet

Therapeutic Actions
This patent formula is used to treat liver cancer; traditional Chinese medicine uses it to treat cancerous tumors, including sarcomas. It invigorates the blood, resolves toxins, softens hardness and stops pain.

Packaged
In box of one hundred tablets.

Dosage
Take four to six tablets, three times per day.

Treatment Note
TCM's use of this formula is typically for a minimum of six months; studies indicate longer use generated a more effective treatment.

Caution
Self-treating cancer is not recommended without competent Western medical evaluation and guidance.

🍁

MALNUTRITION

A diet deficient in carbohydrates is almost inevitably deficient in protein as well. Protein-calorie deficiency is known as malnutrition. Although this deficiency is seen in people who live in abject poverty in the U.S., it is most often seen in people in so-called third world nations as a result of poverty and famine. In Western societies, deficiency of nutrients is usually associated with a disorder of the digestive system, such as celiac sprue, Crohns disease, or pernicious anemia.

Inadequate intake of protein and calories may also occur in people who restrict their diet in an attempt to lose weight, or due to a loss of interest in food associated with alcohol and drug abuse.

Chinese herbal medicine does successfully treat malnutrition by focusing on herbal formulas that increase energy levels, stimulate the appetite, and improve functioning of the digestive system, stop diarrhea and constipation. For optimum results the user is advised to limit alcohol and drug use.

The herbal prescription that follows can be effectively used to treat malnutrition. For this next prescription, I will provide its unique processing instructions and therapeutic action.

RAW HERB FORMULA
Xiao Jian Zhong Tang
Minor Construct the Middle Decoction

Therapeutic Actions
This prescription is used to treat malnutrition; it is very effective for stimulating appetite and treating malnutrition.

Preparation
Traditionally, this formula was used in the raw form to prepare a decoction; however, for those who have not developed the taste for harsh teas, we suggest the user have the ingredients ground into a fine powder by his/her herb supplier, and then store the powder in a brown or amber glass bottle with a lid. Store it in a cool environment free of sunlight and moisture until needed — do not refrigerate.

*Preparation Notes
The herb Yi Tang should not be cooked. Only after the cooking process is completed should you add this herb to the pot, and stir the brew to allow it to dissolve. Then strain off the herbs. The herb Sheng Jiang

or fresh ginger should not be cooked for longer than five minutes. Do not add it to the herbs being cooked until the last five minutes of preparation time.

Dosage for Tang or Decoction
Drink eight ounces of the warm strained decoction (tea), three times a day as needed.

Dosage for Powder
This formula should be taken twice daily. The powder can be used in several different ways. Make a smoothie, by adding twenty to thirty grams of the powder to eight ounces of juice smoothie, mix well, and drink. If that is an issue we recommend adding twenty to thirty grams of powdered herbs to 00-size capsules. For more detailed instructions, follow the step-by-step guide for preparing a smoothie or capsules discussed in Chapter Five.

Herbal Ingredients

Grams	Chinese Herb	Botanical Name	Common Name
18	Bai Shao 白芍	*Paeonia*	White Peony
4 Pieces	Da Zao 大棗	*Ziziphus Jujuba*	Jujube
9	Gui Zhi 桂枝	*Cinnamomum*	Cinnamon Twigs
9	Sheng Jiang* 生姜	*Zingiber Officinale*	Ginger Sliced
30	Yi Tang* 饴糖	*Sacchrum Granorum*	Maltose
6	Zhi Gan Cao 甘草	*Glycyrrhizae*	Licorice

Contraindication
This formula should not be used by patients who have intestinal parasites.

Treatment Note
TCM's use of this formula is typically for a minimum of three months; studies indicate longer use generated a more effective treatment.

NAUSEA

Nausea is simply the sensation of feeling like you need to vomit; although nausea may occur independently of vomiting, generally speaking the causes are the same. Nausea is primarily a symptom of a hangover either from excessive alcohol or drug use.

Chinese herbal medicine does successfully treat nausea by focusing on herbal formulas that settle the stomach, and relieve heartburn, bloating, belching, abdominal cramping, vomiting and diarrhea.

All of the herbal prescriptions that follow can be effectively used to treat nausea. For each prescription, I will provide its unique usage instructions and therapeutic action.

PATENT HERB FORMULAS
Bao Ji Wan
Po Chi Pills

Therapeutic Actions
This patent formula is used to treat the symptoms of a hangover with nausea or heartburn; including bloating, stomach cramping, vomiting, and diarrhea.

Caution
Do not use if pregnant.

Packaged
In box containing ten vials of pills.

Dosage
Take the full contents of one to two vials up to three times daily. In extreme cases you may take an additional vial, making a full dose three vials taken three times daily.

Kang Ning Wan

Pill Curing

Therapeutic Actions

This patent formula is used to treat the symptoms of a hangover with nausea; including belching, vomiting, and abdominal cramping.

Caution

Do not use during pregnancy.

Packaged

In box containing ten vials.

Dosage

Take the full contents of one to two vials up to three times daily.

🍁

NEUROPATHY

Neuropathy is a very complex disease with inflammation, or damage to the peripheral nerves, which connect to the central nervous system, the sense organs, muscles, glands, and internal organs. Symptoms caused by neuropathies include numbness, tingling, pain, or muscle weakness, depending on the nerves affected. In some cases of neuropathy there is no obvious or detectable cause. Among the many specific causes are diabetes, dietary deficiencies (particularly of B vitamins), persistent alcohol consumption, and metabolic upset such as uremia. Other causes include leprosy, lead poisoning, or poisoning by drugs. Nerves may become acutely inflamed after a viral infection such as Guillian Barre Syndrome.

Neuropathies may result from autoimmune disorders such as rheumatoid arthritis, systemic lupus, erythematosus, or periaperitis nodosa. In these disorders there is often damage to the blood vessels supplying the nerves. Neuropathies may occur secondarily to malignant tumors such as lung cancer, or with lymphomas, and leukemia. Finally, there is a group of inherited neuropathies, the most common being peroneal muscular atrophy.

The symptoms of neuropathy depend on whether it affects mainly sensory nerve fibers or motor nerve fibers. Damage to sensory nerve fibers can cause numbness and tingling, sensations of cold, or pain that usually starts in the hands and feet and spreads toward the center of the body. Damage to motor fibers can cause muscle weakness and muscle wasting.

Damage to nerves of the autonomic nervous system can cause blurred vision impaired or the absence of sweating, episodes of faintness associated with a fall in blood pressure, and disturbance of gastric, intestinal, bladder and sexual functioning. Some neuropathies are linked with particular symptoms. An example is the very painful neuropathies that can arise in diabetes and alcohol dependence.

Chinese herbal treatment is aimed at the underlying cause. For example, in cases of diabetes, scrupulous attention to the control of blood sugar levels affords the best chance for relief. Many people with neuropathy may need to stop drinking alcohol, or, if a nutritional deficiency has been diagnosed, vitamins such as thiamine (vitamin B) are usually prescribed. If treatment is successful and the cell bodies of the damaged nerve cells have not been destroyed, a full recovery is possible.

All of the herbal prescriptions that follow can be effectively used to treat neuropathy. For each prescription, I will provide its unique processing instructions and therapeutic action.

RAW HERB FORMULAS
Huang Qi Gui Zhi Wu Wu Tang

Astragalus and Cinnamon Twig Five-Substance Decoction

Therapeutic Actions
This prescription is used to treat neuropathy; it relieves numbness of the nerves to the extremities, shoulders, neck and shoulder pain, muscle paralysis, and facial paralysis.

Preparation

Traditionally, this formula was used in the raw form to prepare a decoction; however, for those who have not developed the taste for harsh teas, we suggest the user have the ingredients ground into a fine powder by his/her herb supplier, and then store the powder in a brown or amber glass bottle with a lid. Store it in a cool environment free of sunlight and moisture until needed — do not refrigerate.

*Preparation Note

The herb Sheng Jiang or fresh ginger should not be cooked for longer than five minutes. Do not add it to the herbs being cooked until the last five minutes of preparation time.

Dosage for Tang or Decoction

Drink four ounces of the warm strained decoction (tea), three times a day as needed.

Dosage for Powder

This formula should be taken twice daily. The powder can be used in several different ways. Make a smoothie, by adding twenty to thirty grams of the powder to eight ounces of juice smoothie, mix well, and drink. If that is an issue we recommend adding twenty to thirty grams of the powdered herbs to 00-size capsules. For more detailed instructions, follow the step-by-step guide for preparing a smoothie or capsules discussed in Chapter Five.

Herbal Ingredients

Grams	Chinese Herb	Botanical Name	Common Name
9	Bai Shao 白芍	*Paeonia*	White Peony
4 Pieces	Da Zao 大棗	*Ziziphus Jujuba*	Jujube
9	Gui Zhi 桂枝	*Cinnamomum*	Cinnamon Twigs
12	Huang Qi 黄芪	*Astragalus*	Milkvetch Root
12	Sheng Jiang* 生姜	*Zingiber Officinale*	Ginger Sliced

Treatment Note

TCM's use of this formula is typically for a minimum of three months; studies indicate longer use generated a more effective treatment.

Tao Hong Si Wu Tang

Four-Substance Decoction with Safflower and Peach Pit

Therapeutic Actions

This prescription is used to treat diabetic neuropathy; it relieves the symptoms of diabetic neuropathy including nerve pain.

Preparation

Traditionally, this formula was used in the raw form to prepare a decoction; however, for those who have not developed the taste for harsh teas, we suggest the user have the ingredients ground into a fine powder by his/her herb supplier, and then store the powder in a brown or amber glass bottle with a lid. Store it in a cool environment free of sunlight and moisture until needed — do not refrigerate.

Dosage for Tang or Decoction

Drink four ounces of the warm strained decoction (tea), three times a day as needed.

Dosage for Powder

This formula should be taken twice daily. The powder can be taken in several different ways. Make a smoothie, by adding twenty to thirty grams of the powder to eight ounces of juice smoothie, mix well, and drink. If that is an issue we recommend adding twenty to thirty grams of the powdered herbs to 00-size capsules. For more detailed instructions, follow the step-by-step guide for preparing a smoothie or capsules discussed in Chapter Five.

Herbal Ingredients

Grams	Chinese Herb	Botanical Name	Common Name
10	Bai Shao 白芍	*Paeonia*	White Peony
8	Chuan Xiong 川芎	*Ligusticum*	Cnidium
12	Dang Gui 當歸	*Angelica*	Angelica
9	Dang Shen 党参	*Codonoposis*	Codonopsis
6	Gou Qi Zi 枸杞子	*Lycii Fructus*	Wolfberry
4	Hong Hua 紅花	*Carthamus*	Carthamus
9	Huang Jing 黃精	*Polygonati*	Solomon's Seal
9	Huang Qi 黄芪	*Astragalus*	Milkvetch
15	Shu Di Huang 熟地黃	*Rehmanniae Preparata*	Rehmannia Cooked
6	Tao Ren 桃仁	*Prunus Persica*	Peach Seed

Contraindications

Do not use this formula if you are pregnant. Use with caution if you have digestive weakness and/or menstrual disorders.

Treatment Note

TCM's use of this formula is typically for a minimum of three months; studies indicate longer use generated a more effective treatment.

PATENT HERB FORMULAS

Bu Yang Huan Wu Great Yang Restoration Teapills

Tonify Yang Return Five Decoction Pills

Therapeutic Actions

This patent formula is used to treat peripheral neuropathy; it relieves numbness of the nerves to the extremities, shoulders, and neck and shoulder pain.

Cautions

Do not use if pregnant. Do not use in acute cases of cerebral hemorrhage.

Packaged

In bottle of two hundred pills.

Dosage

Take eight pills, three times per day. Dosage can be increase to twelve pills, if needed.

Hua Tuo Zai Zao Wan

Hua Tuo Restorative Pills

Therapeutic Actions

This patent formula is used to treat neuropathy; it relieves numbness of the nerves to the extremities, shoulders, and neck and shoulder pain.

Caution

Do not use if pregnant.

Packaged

In box of five hundred small pills packaged in ten smaller boxes; each vial contains eight grams of herbal pills; take one-half vial twice daily.

Dosage

Take one vial daily split in one half, take half in the a.m. the other half in the evening. Dosage can be increase to one full vial in the am and one full vial in the evening, if needed.

Xiao Huo Luo Dan

Minor Invigorate Lou Channel Elixir Pills

Therapeutic Actions

This patent formula is used to treat neuropathy; it relieves numbness of the nerves to the extremities, shoulders, and neck and shoulder pain.

Caution

Do not use if pregnant.

Packaged

In bottle of two hundred pills.

Dosage

Take eight pills, three times per day. Dosage can be increase to twelve pills, if needed.

✤

OVERDOSE

To overdose is to take an excessive amount of a drug which may have a toxic effect that is harmful to certain organs in the body.

Successful Chinese medical treatment of overdose depends on the use of Chinese herbal formulas that drain the toxins out of the body and regulate normal functioning of the body. For optimum effectiveness, it is highly recommended that the user discontinue drugs and alcohol; if this is carried out, full recovery without any permanent damage is possible.

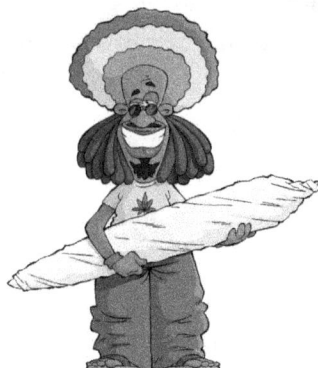

Caution

An overdose can be life-threatening; therefore it is advisable that you seek emergency care at a local hospital.

The herbal prescription that follows can be effectively used to treat overdose. For this next prescription, I will provide its unique processing instructions and therapeutic action.

RAW HERB FORMULA
Tiao Wei Cheng Qi Tang
Regulate the Stomach and Order the Chi Decoction

Therapeutic Actions
This prescription is used to treat drug overdose; it drains toxins (excessive heat) and accumulations out of the body, permitting the body to return to normal function.

Preparation
Traditionally, this formula was used in the raw form to prepare a decoction; however, for those who have not developed the taste for harsh teas, we suggest the user have the ingredients ground into a fine powder by his/her herb supplier, and then store the powder in a brown or amber glass bottle with a lid.

Store it in a cool environment free of sunlight and moisture until needed — do not refrigerate.

*Decoction Preparation Note
One of the herbs in this prescription Mang Xiao should not be cooked, add it at the end of the cooking process just before straining. Stir it well and allow it to dissolve, and then strain off all the herbs.

*Dosage Note
The gram weight to be used in this formula is listed with a minimum/ maximum range. This prescription should be prepared by using the lower dosage and only increase dosage to achieve stronger results when needed.

Dosage for Tang or Decoction
Drink four ounces of the warm strained decoction (tea), as needed.

Dosage for Powder

This formula should be taken once daily. The powder can be taken in several different ways. Make a smoothie, by adding twenty to thirty grams of the powder to eight ounces of juice smoothie, mix well, and drink. If that is an issue we recommend adding twenty to thirty grams of the powdered herbs to 00-size capsules. For more detailed instructions, follow the step-by-step guide for preparing a smoothie or capsules discussed in Chapter Five.

Herbal Ingredients

Grams	Chinese Herb	Botanical Name	Common Name
12	Da Huang 大黃	*Rheum Palmatum*	Rhubarb Root
9-12*	Mang Xiao* 芒硝	*Natrii Sulfas*	Sodium Sulfate
6	Zhi Gan Cao 甘草	*Glycyrrhizae*	Licorice

Caution

Because overdose can be life-threatening, it is advisable to seek emergency care at a local hospital.

🍁

PANCREATITIS

Inflammation of the pancreas is often referred to as a drunk's disease because of its association with excess alcohol consumption. There are two forms of pancreatitis, acute and chronic. In acute pancreatitis the gland usually returns to normal after a single episode; however, in chronic pancreatitis, there is permanent damage to the structure and the function of the pancreas due to persistent inflammation, which causes fibrosis (the formation of fibrous scar tissue) in the gland.

Acute pancreatitis produces a sudden attack of severe upper abdominal pain, often accompanied by nausea and vomiting. The pain may spread to the back, and is made worse by movement; sitting up may relieve it. An attack, which usually lasts for about forty-eight hours, is accompanied by the release of pancreatic enzymes into the blood. Measurement of these enzymes is an important diagnostic test. Ultrasound or CT scanning of the abdomen may also be performed.

Chronic pancreatitis, which usually produces the same symptoms as the acute form, can have several different causes such as: viral infection, mumps, an excess of iron in the body (hemochromatosis), or certain drugs, namely tetracycline. Nevertheless, the most common cause is overindulgence in alcohol. Chronic pancreatitis may also cause insufficient insulin production resulting in Diabetes Mellitus.

If recurrent or chronic pancreatitis causes severe damage to the gland, hypotension (low blood pressure), failure of the heart, kidneys, respiratory system, and ascites (accumulation of fluid in the abdomen) may occur. In some cases cysts or abscesses may develop in the damaged gland.

Successful Chinese herbal treatment for pancreatitis focuses on resolving damp heat (infection), stimulating normal insulin production and nourishing the spleen, stomach and liver. Depending on the level of damage to the pancreas full recovery is possible; however, limiting the use of alcohol and drugs is highly recommended.

All of the herbal prescriptions that follow can be effectively used to treat pancreatitis. For each prescription, I will provide its unique processing instructions and therapeutic action.

RAW HERB FORMULA
Da Cheng Qi Tang
Major Order the Qi Decoction

Therapeutic Actions
This formula is used to treat pancreatitis; with symptoms including abdominal pain, nausea, vomiting and constipation.

Preparation

Traditionally, this formula was used in the raw form to prepare a decoction; however, for those who have not developed the taste for harsh teas, we suggest the user have the ingredients ground into a fine powder by his/her herb supplier, and then store the powder in a brown or amber glass bottle with a lid. Store it in a cool environment free of sunlight and moisture until needed — do not refrigerate.

*Decoction Preparation Note

One of the herbs in this prescription Mang Xiao should not be cooked, add it at the end of the cooking process just before straining. Stir it well and allow it to dissolve, and then strain off all the herbs.

Dosage for Tang or Decoction

Drink four ounces of the warm strained decoction (tea), as needed.

Dosage for Powder

This formula should be taken once daily. The powder can be used in several different ways. Make a smoothie, by adding twenty to thirty grams of the powder to eight ounces of juice smoothie, mix well, and drink. If that is an issue we recommend adding twenty to thirty grams of the powdered herbs to 00-size capsules. For more detailed instructions, follow the step-by-step guide for preparing a smoothie or capsules discussed in Chapter Five.

Herbal Ingredients

Grams	Chinese Herb	Botanical Name	Common Name
12	Da Huang 大黄	*Rheum Palmatum*	Rhubarb
24	Hou Po 厚朴	*Magnolia*	Magnolia
6	Mang Xiao* 芒硝	*Natrii Sulfas*	Sodium Sulfate
12	Zhi Shi 炒枳實	*Citrus Aurantium*	Bitter Orange

Contraindications

Do not use if pregnant. Do not use for geriatric patients.

PATENT HERB FORMULA
Da Chai Hu Wan

Major Bupleurum Pills

Therapeutic Actions

This patent formula is used to treat pancreatitis with symptoms of vomiting, nausea, abdominal pain, with bloating and constipation.

Caution

Do not use during pregnancy.

Packaged

In bottle of two hundred pills.

Dosage

Take eight pills three times daily.

🍁

PEPTIC ULCER

When an area of the digestive system becomes raw, a sore develops that is constantly bathed by gastric acid, which will create a painful burning sensation—a peptic ulcer. A peptic ulcer is a common side-effect of alcoholism.

The ulcer can occur in the esophagus, stomach or duodenum. Although many people found to have peptic ulcers have no symptoms, typically sufferers will experience a burning, gnawing pain in the abdomen, which sometimes wakes them at night. Psychological stress may also play a role in making an existing ulcer worse.

In some cases complications such as bleeding can develop, which can result in vomiting blood and having bowel movements that are very dark or black -- an indication of blood in the feces. Chronic blood loss can lead to blood deficiency and anemia. Common symptoms of anemia are: fatigue or a general lack of energy, pale complexion and shortness of breath.

Rarely, an ulcer may penetrate the back wall of the digestive tract causing pain that spreads to the sufferer's back.

If the affected area is on the front wall of the duodenum, the leaking digestive juices may cause peritonitis (inflammation of the abdominal lining) producing sudden severe abdominal pain. In a small number of cases gastric ulcers can be malignant and should be removed as soon as they are diagnosed.

Self-help methods include:
- Avoid smoking
- Avoid drinking alcohol, coffee, and tea
- Avoid using aspirin and non-steroidal anti-inflammatory drugs
- Eat several small meals at regular intervals

According to traditional Chinese medical theory, peptic ulcers are a result of excess dampness (in Chinese medicine this is any kind of turbidity (mucus, phlegm, etc.)), acidity, and heat in the digestive system. Herbal formulas that treat peptic ulcers resolve that dampness and neutralize acidity by using ingredients that re-establish the acid/alkaline balance, and extinguish the heat that causes the burning sensation, through its use of cool herbs that regenerate tissue and heal sores. Additional symptoms such as: belching, feeling bloated, nausea, weight loss and vomiting, are also resolved when the Chinese herbs address the chemical balance (such as acid/alkaline balance) and the stomach is harmonized. Once treatment begins, the patient should experience some relief and expect to completely recover within six to eight weeks. If the ulcer fails to respond, surgery may be the only option.

All of the herbal prescriptions that follow can be effectively used to treat ulcers. For each prescription, I will provide its unique processing instructions and therapeutic action.

RAW HERB FORMULA
Huang Qi Jian Zhong Tang
Astragalus Decoction to Construct the Middle

Therapeutic Actions
This formula is used to treat peptic ulcer, it will harmonize the center (the digestive system), relieve pain, reduce acidity and bloating, and stop bleeding.

Preparation
Traditionally, this formula was used in the raw form to prepare a decoction; however, for those who have not developed the taste for harsh teas, we suggest the user have the ingredients ground into a fine powder by his/her herb supplier, and then store the powder in a brown or amber glass bottle with a lid. Store it in a cool environment free of sunlight and moisture until needed — do not refrigerate.

*Preparation Notes
The herb Yi Tang should not be cooked. Only after the cooking process is completed should you add this herb to the pot, and stir the brew to allow it to dissolve. Then strain off the herbs. The herb Sheng Jiang or fresh ginger should not be cooked for longer than five minutes. Do not add it to the herbs being cooked until the last five minutes of preparation time.

Dosage for Tang or Decoction

Drink four to eight ounces of the warm strained decoction (tea), daily as needed.

Dosage for Powder

This formula should be taken once daily. The powder can be used in several different ways. Make a smoothie, by adding twenty to thirty grams of the powder to eight ounces of juice smoothie, mix well, and drink. If that is an issue we recommend adding twenty to thirty grams of the powdered herbs to 00-size capsules. For more detailed instructions, follow the step-by-step guide for preparing a smoothie or capsules discussed in Chapter Five.

Herbal Ingredients

Grams	Chinese Herb	Botanical Name	Common Name
6	Bai Ji 白芨	Bletilla Striata	Hyacinth
18	Bai Shao 白芍	Paeonia	White Peony
6	Chen Pi 陳皮	Citrus Reticulate	Tangerine Peel
4 Pieces	Da Zao 大棗	Ziziphus Jujuba	Jujube
9	Gui Zhi 桂枝	Cinnamomum	Cinnamon Twigs
9	Hai Piao Xiao 乌贼骨	Sepiaella Maindroni	Cuttlefish Bone
12	Huang Qi 黄芪	Astragalus	Milkvetch
6	Mai Ya 麦芽	Hordeum Vulgare	Barley Sprout
6	San Qi 三七	Notoginseng	Pseudoginseng
9	Sheng Jiang* 生姜	Zingiber Officinale	Ginger Sliced
9	Wa Leng Zi 瓦楞子	Arca Subcrenata	Ark Shell
9	Yan Hu Suo 延胡索	Corydalis	Corydalis
30	Yi Tang* 饴糖	Sacchrum Granorum	Maltose
6	Zhi Gan Cao 甘草	Glycyrrhizae	Licorice
6	Zhi Ke 枳殼	Citrus Aurantium	Bitter Orange

PATENT HERB FORMULA
Zhong Guo Zhi Wei Bao
China Treat Stomach Treasure

Therapeutic Actions
This patent formula is used to treat peptic ulcer. It will stop bleeding, reduce acidity, clear abdominal heat, and reduce inflammation. This formula is used to treat both bleeding and non-bleeding ulcers.

Caution
This formula is most effective when used for short term acute attacks; do not use long-term.

Packaged
In box of ten vials.

Dosage
Take one-half-vial, two times daily.

❧

PHLEBITIS

Phlebitis is an inflammation of a vein — that's often accompanied by formation of a blood clot. The medical name for this condition is thrombophlebitis.

Thrombophlebitis can occur after minor injury to a vein (such as after an injection) and is particularly common in intravenous drug users.

There is obvious swelling and redness along the affected segment of the vein, which is extremely tender to the touch. Fever and malaise often occur.

Serious complications are uncommon, although sometimes more serious clot formation develops in deeper veins (deep vein thrombosis).

Normally treatment involves providing gentle support using a crepe bandage along with taking anti-inflammatory Chinese herbal formulas and sometimes antibiotic herbs are also taken if infection of the vein is suspected.

All of the herbal prescriptions that follow can be effectively used to treat phlebitis. For each prescription, I will provide its unique processing instructions and therapeutic action.

RAW HERB FORMULAS
Si Miao Yong An Tang
Four-Valiant Decoction for Well-Being

Therapeutic Actions
This prescription is used to treat phlebitis; it relieves the pain and inflammation in the veins of the neck, legs and arms.

Preparation (for internal use)
Traditionally, this formula was used in the raw form to prepare a decoction; however, for those who have not developed the taste for harsh teas, we suggest the user have the ingredients ground into a fine powder by his/ her herb supplier, and then store the powder in a brown or amber glass bottle with a lid. Store it in a cool environment free of sunlight and moisture until needed — do not refrigerate.

*Dosage Note
The gram weight to be used in this formula is listed with a minimum/ maximum range. This prescription should be prepared by using the lower dosage and only increase dosage to achieve stronger results when needed.

Dosage for Tang or Decoction (for internal use)
Drink eight ounces of the warm strained decoction (tea), three times a day as needed.

Dosage for Powder (for internal use)

This formula should be taken twice daily. The powder can be taken in several different ways. Make a smoothie, by adding twenty to thirty grams of the powder to eight ounces of juice smoothie, mix well, and drink. If that is an issue we recommend adding twenty to thirty grams of the powdered herbs to 00-size capsules. For more detailed instructions, follow the step-by-step guide for preparing a smoothie or capsules discussed in Chapter Five.

Treatment Note (for external use)

This prescription can be used "internally" (as described above) or it can be applied to the skin for "external" pain relief. To make an external wrap prepare a compress. An herbal compress is made by first decocting the herbs. After the tea is made, the herbs can either be strained and discarded, or left in the pot and allowed to cool. Leaving the herbs in the pot, I should mention, increases the potency of the herbal mixture. Once prepared, the decocted tea can be re-used for approximately five to seven days by simply keeping the pot covered and reheating when needed. It is not necessary to boil the herbal brew a second time as long as you keep the pot covered and reheat the decoction every day, it should not become rancid. However, if you are concerned about maintaining the freshness of the herbal tea, then I suggest you store it in a closed glass jar in the refrigerator and reheat – it should be usable for up to two weeks when refrigerated. The compress is prepared by soaking sterile surgical gauze or some other sterile soft cotton material in the warm herbal tea, then the excess fluid is wrung out, and the cotton material is applied to the injured area. When making a compress the cotton material should be saturated with the fluid, but not dripping. Then wrap the area with a warm towel or blanket to promote sweating. Repeat the process as needed.

Herbal Ingredients

Grams	Chinese Herb	Botanical Name	Common Name
15–30*	Dang Gui 當歸	*Angelica*	Angelica
10–15*	Gan Cao 甘草	*Glycyrrhiza Uralensis*	Licorice
30–90*	Jin Yin Hua 金银花	*Lonicera*	Honeysuckle
30–90*	Xuan Shen 玄参	*Scrophularia*	Figwort

Contraindication

Avoid scratching the affected area during treatment.

Xue Fu Zhu Yu Tang

Drive out Stasis in the Mansion of Blood Decoction

Therapeutic Actions

This prescription is used to treat phlebitis; it relieves inflammation of the neck, leg and arm veins of redness and swelling, pain and inflammation.

Preparation

Traditionally, this formula was used in the raw form to prepare a decoction; however, for those who have not developed the taste for harsh teas, we suggest the user have the ingredients ground into a fine powder by his/her herb supplier, and then store the powder in a brown or amber glass bottle with a lid. Store it in a cool environment free of sunlight and moisture until needed — do not refrigerate.

Dosage for Tang or Decoction

Drink four ounces of the warm strained decoction (tea), three times a day as needed.

Dosage for Powder

This formula should be taken twice daily. The powder can be taken in several different ways. Make a smoothie, by adding twenty to thirty grams of the powder to eight ounces of juice smoothie, mix well, and drink.

If that is an issue we recommend adding twenty to thirty grams of the powdered herbs to 00-size capsules. For more detailed instructions, follow the step-by-step guide for preparing a smoothie or capsules discussed in Chapter Five.

Herbal Ingredients

Grams	Chinese Herb	Botanical Name	Common Name
3	Chai Hu 柴胡	*Bupleurum*	Bupleurum
6	Chi Shao 赤芍	*Paeonia Veitchii*	Red Peony
9	Chuan Niu Xi 川牛膝	*Cyathula*	Cyathula
4.5	Chuan Xiong 川芎	*Ligusticum*	Cnidium
9	Dang Gui 當歸	*Angelica*	Angelica
6	Gan Cao 甘草	*Glycyrrhiza Uralensis*	Licorice
9	Hong Hua 紅花	*Carthamus*	Carthamus
4.5	Jie Geng 桔梗	*Platycodon*	Platycodon
9	Shu Di Huang 熟地黄	*Rehmanniae Preparata*	Rehmannia Cooked
12	Tao Ren 桃仁	*Prunus Persica*	Peach Seed
6	Zhi Ke 枳殼	*Citrus Aurantium*	Bitter Orange

Contraindication

Do not use this formula if you are pregnant.

PATENT HERB FORMULAS
Raw Tienchi Tablets

Yunnan Province Specially Produced Notoginseng Tablets

Therapeutic Actions

This patent formula is used to treat phlebitis; it relieves pain and inflammation of a vein.

Caution

Do not use if pregnant.

Packaged
In box of thirty six pills, each contains 0.5 gram of herb.

Dosage
Take two to four tablets, three times per day.

Xin Mai Ling
Miraculously Effective Pills for Coronary Circulation

Therapeutic Actions
This prescription is used to treat phlebitis; it relieves the pain and inflammation in the veins of the neck, legs and arms.

Caution
Do not use if pregnant, or if taking blood thinners as clotting time can be significantly reduced.

Packaged
In box of thirty six pills.

Dosage
Take three pills three times per day. In severe cases dosage can be increased to four to five pills.

🍁

PNEUMONIA

Pneumonia is an inflammation of the lungs due to infection; there are two main types of pneumonia, lobar pneumonia and bronchopneumonia. In lobar pneumonia one lobe initially is affected. In bronchopneumonia, inflammation starts in the bronchi and bronchioles (airways) and then spreads to affect patches of tissue in one or both lungs.

Most cases of pneumonia are caused by viruses or bacteria. Rarely

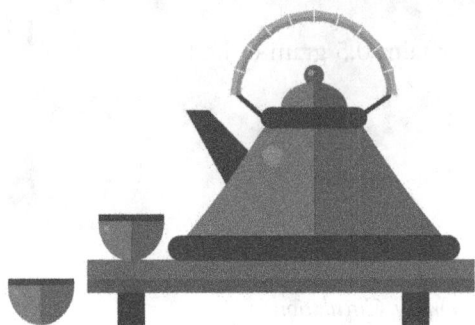

pneumonia may be due to a different type of organism, such as fungi, yeasts, or protozoa. These types usually only occur in people with immunodeficiency disorders such as AIDS.

Symptoms and signs typically include shortness of breath, and a cough that produces yellow-green sputum and occasionally blood.

Chest pain that is worse when inhaling may occur because of pleurisy (inflammation of the membrane lining the lungs and chest cavity).

Potential complications include pleural effusion (fluid around the lungs), empyema (pus in the pleural cavity) and rarely an abscess in the lung.

Successful treatment using Chinese herbal medicine focuses on relieving the symptoms of pneumonia, including but not limited to fever, chronic cough, and excessive inflammation of the lungs, chest pain, and sore throat.

All of the herbal prescriptions that follow can be effectively used to treat pneumonia. For each prescription, I will provide its unique processing instructions and therapeutic action.

RAW HERB FORMULAS
Liang Ge San
Cool the Diaphragm Powder

Therapeutic Actions
This prescription is used to treat pneumonia; it relieves the symptoms of pneumonia such as an aversion to cold, fever, cough and chest pain.

Preparation

Traditionally, this formula was used in the raw form to make a decoction; however, for those who have not developed the taste for harsh teas, we suggest the user have the ingredients ground into a fine powder by his/her herb supplier, and then store the powder in a brown or amber glass bottle with a lid. Store it in a cool environment free of sunlight and moisture until needed — do not refrigerate.

*Preparation Note

The Bo He should not be cooked with the rest of this formula. After finishing the cooking process, add in the Bo He, stir well, and then steep the decoction for fifteen minutes, and then strain off the herbs.

Dosage for Tang or Decoction

Drink four to eight ounces of the warm strained decoction (tea), one-two times a day as needed.

Dosage for Powder

This formula should be taken one to two times daily. The powder can be used in several different ways. Make a smoothie, by adding twenty to thirty grams of the powder to eight ounces of juice smoothie, mix well, and drink. If that is an issue we recommend adding twenty to thirty grams of the powdered herbs to 00-size capsules. For more detailed instructions, follow the step-by-step guide for preparing a smoothie or capsules discussed in Chapter Five.

Herbal Ingredients

Grams	Chinese Herb	Botanical Name	Common Name
5	Bo He* 薄荷	*Mentha*	Mint
9	Da Huang 大黃	*Rheum Palmatum*	Rhubarb Root
3	Feng Mi 蜂蜜	*Apis Cerana*	Honey
9	Gan Cao 甘草	*Glycyrrhiza Uralensis*	Licorice
5	Huang Qin 黃芩	*Schutellaria*	Baikal Skullcap
18	Lian Qiao 连翘	*Forsythia*	Forsythia
9	Po Xiao 芒硝	*Sal Glauberis*	Sodium Sulfate
5	Zhi Zi 栀子	*Gardenia*	Gardenia
3	Zhu Ye 苦竹叶	*Phyllostachys*	Bamboo Leaves

Qing Fei Tang

Clear the Lung Decoction

Therapeutic Actions

This prescription is used to treat pneumonia; it relieves the symptoms of pneumonia with chronic cough, excessive inflammation in the lungs, severe cough, phlegm, sore and itch throat, and hoarseness.

Preparation

Traditionally, this formula was used in the raw form to prepare a decoction; however, for those who have not developed the taste for harsh teas, we suggest the user have the ingredients ground into a fine powder by his/her herb supplier, and then store the powder in a brown or amber glass bottle with a lid. Store it in a cool environment free of sunlight and moisture until needed — do not refrigerate.

Dosage for Tang or Decoction

Drink four ounces of the warm strained decoction (tea), three times a day as needed.

Dosage for Powder

This formula should be taken twice daily. The powder can be used in several different ways. Make a smoothie, by adding twenty to thirty grams of the powder to eight ounces of juice smoothie, mix well, and drink. If that is an issue we recommend adding twenty to thirty grams of the powdered herbs to 00-size capsules. For more detailed instructions, follow the step-by-step guide for preparing a smoothie or capsules discussed in Chapter Five.

Herbal Ingredients

Grams	Chinese Herb	Botanical Name	Common Name
3	Chen Pi 陳皮	*Citrus Reticulate*	Tangerine Peel
2.1	Dang Gui 當歸	*Angelica*	Angelica
3	Fu Ling 茯苓	*Poria Cocos*	Tuckahoe
0.9	Gan Cao 甘草	*Glycyrrhiza Uralensis*	Licorice
4.5	Huang Qin 黃芩	*Schutellaria*	Baikal Skullcap
3	Jie Geng 桔梗	*Platycodon*	Platycodon
2.1	Ku Xing Ren 杏仁	*Prunus Armeniaca*	Apricot Seed
2.1	Mai Men Dong 麦冬	*Ophiopogon*	Winter Wheat
3	Sang Bai Pi 桑白皮	*Morus Alba*	Mulberry Bark
2.1	Tian Men Dong 天門冬	*Asparagus*	Asparagus
7 Pieces	Wu Wei Zi 五味子	*Schisandra*	Schizandra
3	Zhe Bai Mu 浙貝毌	*Fritillaria*	Fritillary Bulb
2.1	Zhi Zi 梔子	*Gardenia*	Gardenia
3	Zhu Ru 竹茹	*Bambusa Breviflora*	Bamboo

Shen Su Yin

Ginseng and Perilla Leaf Decoction

Therapeutic Actions

This prescription is used to treat pneumonia; it relieves the symptoms of pneumonia including phlegm retention, severe cough, fever, headache, nasal obstruction, cough with profuse sputum, and fullness of the chest, fatigue, lethargy and shortness of breath.

Preparation

Traditionally, this formula was used in the raw form to prepare a decoction; however, for those who have not developed the taste for harsh teas, we suggest the user have the ingredients ground into a fine powder by his/ her herb supplier, and then store the powder in a brown or amber glass bottle with a lid. Store it in a cool environment free of sunlight and moisture until needed — do not refrigerate.

Dosage for Tang or Decoction

Drink four ounces of the warm strained decoction (tea), three times a day as needed.

Dosage for Powder

This formula should be taken twice daily. The powder can be taken in several different ways. Make a smoothie, by adding twenty to thirty grams of the powder to eight ounces of juice smoothie, mix well, and drink. If that is an issue we recommend adding twenty to thirty grams of the powdered herbs to 00-size capsules. For more detailed instructions, follow the step-by-step guide for preparing a smoothie or capsules discussed in Chapter Five.

Herbal Ingredients

Grams	Chinese Herb	Botanical Name	Common Name
6	Ban Xia 半夏	*Pinellia Ternata*	Half Summer
4	Chen Pi 陳皮	*Citrus Reticulate*	Tangerine Peel
6	Fu Ling 茯苓	*Poria Cocos*	Tuckahoe
4	Gan Cao 甘草	*Glycyrrhiza Uralensis*	Licorice
6	Ge Gen 葛根	*Puerariae*	Kudzu
4	Jie Geng 桔梗	*Platycodon*	Platycodon
4	Mu Xiang 木香	*Aucklandiae*	Costus
6	Qian Hu 前胡	*Peucedanum Pracruptorum*	Hog-Fennel
6	Ren Shen 人参	*Ginseng*	Ginseng
4	Zhi Ke 枳殼	*Citrus Aurantium*	Bitter Orange
6	Zi Su Ye 紫蘇	Perilla	Perilla Leaf

SEXUAL DYSFUNCTION

There are basically four types of sexual dysfunction associated with excessive use of alcohol or drugs: loss of sexual desire, arousal disorder (the inability to maintain an erection in men, and for women maintaining arousal during intercourse), difficulty reaching orgasm, and painful intercourse.

In moderation alcohol can increase sexual arousal, and lessen inhibitions, and certain drugs such as marijuana, and amphetamines are known to enhance the sexual experience and intensify orgasm. However, substance abuse like binge drinking and drugging is known to negatively affect sexual behavior, as well as a person's ability to function and experience physical sensations which can diminish sexual pleasure.

Well-known causes of sexual dysfunction are opiates like heroin and oxycontin, tranquilizers like valium, anti-depressants like prozac and barbiturates such as phenobarbital. The following is a list of recreational drugs and their effect on sexual performance:

- **Amphetamines:** Can increase stamina and intensify orgasm. Habitual long term use is associated with ejaculatory disorders; abuse of cocaine is associated with reduction of sexual sensation in both women and men, and reduced sexual performance in men.

- **Anabolic steroids:** Reduce the libido as well as the size of the testicles, and can cause infertility in men. In women steroid use can reduce the sex-drive and masculinize.

- **Ecstasy:** Enhances the libido and can increase sex-drive at the expense of impaired sexual performance (delayed orgasm and erectile dysfunction).

- **Marijuana:** Increases sexual arousal and intensifies orgasm. Heightened sensitivity can cause premature ejaculation.

- **Poppers (alkyl nitrate):** Increase sexual arousal by increasing blood flow to the genitals. If used with sildenafil, it can cause severe lowering of blood pressure.

- **Psycho-stimulants (LSD):** Can increase sexual desire in the short term, but long-term use has been known to have the opposite effect and decrease sex drive.

Chinese medical treatment can cure sexual dysfunction; Chinese herbal medicine focuses on re-establishing normal levels of sexual desire and functioning, including the ability to maintain an erection, maintain seminal fluid and normal ejaculation, or for women maintaining arousal during intercourse. Discontinuing alcohol and drug use is required, and if this is carried out, full recovery is possible.

All of the herbal prescriptions that follow can be effectively used to treat sexual dysfunction. For each prescription, I will provide its unique processing instructions and therapeutic action.

RAW HERB FORMULAS
Long Dan Xie Gan Tang
Gentiana Decoction to Drain the Liver

Therapeutic Actions
This formula is used to treat the symptoms of sexual dysfunction in males, and treat the inability to ejaculate.

Preparation
Traditionally, this formula was used in the raw form to prepare a decoction; however, for those who have not developed the taste for harsh teas, we suggest the user have the ingredients ground into a fine powder by his/her herb supplier, and then store the powder in a brown or amber glass bottle with a lid. Store it in a cool environment free of sunlight and moisture until needed — do not refrigerate.

Dosage for Tang or Decoction
Drink four ounces of the warm strained decoction (tea), three times a day as needed.

Dosage for Powder
This formula should be taken twice daily. The powder can be used in several

different ways. Make a smoothie, by adding twenty to thirty grams of the powder to eight ounces of juice smoothie, mix well, and drink. If that is an issue we recommend adding twenty to thirty grams of the powdered herbs to 00-size capsules. For more detailed instructions, follow the step-by-step guide for preparing a smoothie or capsules discussed in Chapter Five.

Herbal Ingredients

Grams	Chinese Herb	Botanical Name	Common Name
6	Chai Hu 柴胡	*Bupleurum*	Bupleurum
9	Che Qian Zi 車前子	*Plantago*	Plantago
9	Chuan Mu Tong 川木通	*Clematis Armandii*	Clematis
3	Dang Gui 當歸	*Angelica*	Angelica
6	Gan Cao 甘草	*Glycyrrhiza*	Licorice
9	Hai Piao Xiao 乌贼骨	*Sepiaella*	Cuttlefish Bone
9	Huang Qin 黃芩	*Schutellaria*	Baikal Skullcap
6	Long Dan 龙胆	*Gentiana*	Gentian
10	Qian Cao 茜草	*Rubiae India*	Madder Root
9	Shu Di Huang 熟地黃	*Rehmanniae Preparata*	Rehmannia Cooked
12	Ze Xie 澤瀉	*Alisma Orientalis*	Water Plantain
9	Zhi Mu 知母	*Anemarrhena*	Anemarrhena
9	Zhi Zi 栀子	*Gardenia*	Gardenia

Contraindication

This formula should not be used for those with blood deficiencies.

Fu Tu Dan

Poria and Cuscuta Special Pill

Therapeutic Actions

This formula is used to treat the symptoms of sexual dysfunction in males, such as spermatorrhea, leakage of seminal fluid, and premature ejaculation.

Preparation

Traditionally, this formula was used in the raw form to prepare a decoction;

however, for those who have not developed the taste for harsh teas, we suggest the user have the ingredients ground into a fine powder by his/her herb supplier, and then store the powder in a brown or amber glass bottle with a lid. Store it in a cool environment free of sunlight and moisture until needed — do not refrigerate.

Dosage for Tang or Decoction

Drink four ounces of the warm strained decoction (tea), three times a day as needed.

Dosage for Powder

The powder can be used in several different ways. Make a smoothie, by adding twenty to thirty grams of the powder to eight ounces of juice smoothie, mix well, and drink twice daily. If that is an issue we recommend adding twenty to thirty grams of the powdered herbs to 00-size capsules, and daily dosage is three capsules containing 3 grams each taken three times daily. For more detailed instructions, follow the step-by-step guide for preparing a smoothie or capsules discussed in Chapter Five.

Herbal Ingredients

Grams	Chinese Herb	Botanical Name	Common Name
150	Fu Ling 茯苓	*Poria Cocos*	Tuckahoe
180	Shan Yao 山药	*Dioscorea*	Yam
90	Shi Lian Zi 石莲子	*Sinocrassulae Indicae*	Black Lotus Seed
300	Tu Si Zi 菟絲子	*Cuscuta*	Dodder Seed
210	Wu Wei Zi 五味子	*Schisandra*	Schizandra

PATENT FORMULAS
Kang Wei Ling Pills

Therapeutic Actions

This prescription is used to treat sexual dysfunction. It contains a powerful combination of angelica, licorice and centipede that increases circulation of blood to the genitalia it corrects impotence, premature ejaculation, and it will increase sexual desire.

Packaged

In bottle of one hundred twenty pills.

Dosage

Take ten to fifteen pills, two to three times per day.

Lu Bao Bu Shen Pills

Therapeutic Actions

This prescription is used to treat sexual dysfunction; it is considered by many of the men of China to be an answer to lifelong sexual health. It is a very strong male tonic that will increase sex drive, impotence, premature ejaculation, or the failure to obtain an erection. This tonic nourishes the kidneys and will benefit anyone suffering from diabetes.

Packaged

In bottle of thirty six pills.

Dosage

Take three to four pills, one to two times per day.

❦

SYPHILIS

Syphilis is a sexually transmitted or congenital (existing at birth) infection that was first recorded as a major epidemic in Europe in the last decade of the fifteenth century, following the return of Columbus from his travels in the Americas.

Today, the infection is transmitted almost exclusively by sexual contact. Congenital syphilis, once very common, is now rare. Symptoms of infection usually pass through the following stages:

The Primary Stage

The first symptom is a sore (chancre) that usually appears three to four weeks after contact with an infected person. The chancre is a painless ulcer with a hard wet base that is covered with serum-teeming spirochetes. The usual site is the genitals, but may be the anus, mouth, rectum, or fingers. Often, the sore is inconspicuous and may be missed. The lymph nodes connected with the area containing the chancre become enlarged but not tender. The chancre heals in four to eight weeks.

The Secondary Stage

Occurs six to twelve weeks after infection; the most obvious feature is a skin rash which may be transient, recurrent or may last for months. On white skin, the rash is more conspicuous (pinkish or pale red spots); on black or African American skin the rash is pigmented and appears darker than the normal skin color. The rash is associated with extensive enlargement of the lymph nodes. There is often headache, aches and pains in the bones, loss of appetite, fever, and fatigue. The hair may fall out in clumps, and in moist areas thickened gray or pink patches called condylomata lata may develop—which are highly infectious! The secondary stage may persist for about a year.

The Final Stage

When the infection reaches the next stage called latent, which may last for a few years or the rest of the person's life, the infected person appears normal.

However, about thirty percent of untreated cases eventually proceed to tertiary syphilis. This stage usually starts within ten years of infection, but may appear as early as three years or as late as twenty-five years. The effects are varied. Tissue destruction by a process called gumma-formation, may involve the bones, palate, nasal septum, tongue, skin, or almost any organ of the body. Among the more serious effects are cardiovascular syphilis, which affects the aorta (the main artery of the body) and leads to aneurysm, heart valve disease, with progressive brain damage, and general paralysis.

Successful Chinese medical treatment depends on the use of herbal formulas that focus on treating the infection, abdominal and genital pain and discomfort, and clear up discharge, itch and lower back pain. As with all STD it is advisable to treat all sexual partners to avoid reinfection.

The herbal prescription that follows can be effectively used to treat syphilis. For the following prescription, I will provide its unique processing instructions and therapeutic action.

RAW HERB FORMULA
Long Dan Xie Gan Tang
Gentiana Decoction to Drain the Liver

Therapeutic Actions
This prescription is used to treat gonorrhea; it relieves the symptoms of syphilis, gonorrhea, herpes zoster, and abnormal vaginal discharge.

Preparation
Traditionally, this formula was used in the raw form to prepare a decoction; however, for those who have not developed the taste for harsh teas, we suggest the user have the ingredients ground into a fine powder by his/her herb supplier, and then store the powder in a brown or amber glass bottle with a lid. Store it in a cool environment free of sunlight and moisture until needed — do not refrigerate.

Dosage for Tang or Decoction
Drink four ounces of the warm strained decoction (tea), three times a day as needed.

Dosage for Powder

This formula should be taken twice daily. The powder can be used in several different ways. Make a smoothie, by adding twenty to thirty grams of the powder to eight ounces of juice smoothie, mix well, and drink. If that is an issue we recommend adding twenty to thirty grams of the powdered herbs to 00-size capsules. For more detailed instructions, follow the step-by-step guide for preparing a smoothie or capsules discussed in Chapter Five.

Herbal Ingredients

Grams	Chinese Herb	Botanical Name	Common Name
6	Chai Hu 柴胡	*Bupleurum*	Bupleurum
9	Che Qian Zi 車前子	*Plantago*	Plantago Seed
9	Chuan Mu Tong 川木通	*Clematis Armandii*	Clematis
3	Dang Gui 當歸	*Angelica*	Angelica
6	Gan Cao 甘草	*Glycyrrhiza*	Licorice
9	Hai Piao Xiao 乌贼骨	*Sepiaella*	Cuttlefish Bone
9	Huang Qin 黄芩	*Schutellaria*	Baikal Skullcap
6	Long Dan 龙胆	*Gentiana Scabra*	Gentian
10	Qian Cao 茜草	*Radix Rubiae*	India Madder
9	Shu Di Huang 熟地黃	*Rehmanniae Preparata*	Rehmannia Cooked
12	Ze Xie 澤瀉	*Alisma*	Water Plantain
9	Zhi Mu 知母	*Anemarrhena*	Anemarrhena
9	Zhi Zi 栀子	*Gardenia*	Gardenia

Contraindication

This formula should not be used for those with blood deficiencies.

Note

As with all STD it is advisable to treat all sexual partners to avoid reinfection.

TUBERCULOSIS

Tuberculosis is the disease commonly referred to as TB; aka consumption, which is caused by the bacterium mycobacterium tuberculosis. The disease is also more common in the elderly, people with immune deficiency disorders, diabetics, and alcoholics.

The main symptoms include coughing (sometimes coughing up blood), chest pain, shortness of breath, fever and sweating (especially at night), poor appetite, and weight loss.

There are two types of TB; the more familiar form pulmonary tuberculosis primarily affects the lungs and is spread from person to person by coughing or sneezing. The lesser-known variety, bovine tuberculosis involves the intestines, bones, and other organs and is transmitted through contaminated cow's milk.

The main complications of tuberculosis are pleural effusion (fluid build-up between the lung and the chest wall) and pneumothorax (air between the lung and the chest wall). The incidence of TB is higher in certain racial or social groups -- namely Hispanics, Haitians and Southeast Asians.

Chinese medical treatment successfully treats tuberculosis, using Chinese herbal medicine that focus on relieving the cough, chest pain, shortness of breath, fever, night sweats, lack of appetite, and fluid retention. Taking a break from alcohol and drug use is a good idea, and if this is carried out, full recovery is possible.

All of the herbal prescriptions that follow can be effectively used to treat tuberculosis. For each prescription, I will provide processing instructions and the formula's therapeutic actions.

RAW HERB FORMULAS
Bu Fei Tang
Tonify the Lung Decoction

Therapeutic Actions
Used to treat tuberculosis; and relieve symptoms such as: cough, asthma and pulmonary tuberculosis, lung congestion, wheezing, shortness of breath, chills, spontaneous sweating, and a pale face.

Preparation
Traditionally, this formula was used in the raw form to prepare a decoction; however, for those who have not developed the taste for harsh teas, we suggest the user have the ingredients ground into a fine powder by his/her herb supplier, and then store the powder in a brown or amber glass bottle with a lid. Store it in a cool environment free of sunlight and moisture until needed — do not refrigerate.

Dosage for Tang or Decoction
Drink four ounces of the warm strained decoction (tea), three times a day as needed.

Dosage for Powder
This formula should be taken twice daily. The powder can be used in several different ways. Make a smoothie, by adding twenty to thirty grams of the powder to eight ounces of juice smoothie, mix well, and drink. If that is an issue we recommend adding twenty to thirty grams of the powdered herbs to 00-size capsules. For more detailed instructions, follow the step-by-step guide for preparing a smoothie or capsules discussed in Chapter Five.

Herbal Ingredients

Grams	Chinese Herb	Botanical Name	Common Name
24	Huang Qi 黃芪	*Astragalus*	Milkvetch
9	Ren Shen 人參	*Ginseng*	Ginseng
12	Sang Bai Pi 桑白皮	*Morus Alba*	Mulberry Bark
24	Shu Di Huang 熟地黃	*Rehmanniae Preparata*	Rehmannia Cooked
6	Wu Wei Zi 五味子	*Schisandra*	Schizandra
9	Zi Wan 紫苑	*Asteris*	Tartarian Aster

Jiu Xian San

Nine Immortal Powder

Therapeutic Actions

Used to treat tuberculosis, calm the lungs and stop cough. This formula can be used to treat persistent coughing, wheezing and sweating with fever in chronic bronchitis and pulmonary tuberculosis.

Preparation

Traditionally, this formula was used in the raw form to prepare a decoction; however, for those who have not developed the taste for harsh teas, we suggest the user have the ingredients ground into a fine powder by his/her herb supplier, and then store the powder in a brown or amber glass bottle with a lid. Store it in a cool environment free of sunlight and moisture until needed — do not refrigerate.

*Preparation Note

The herb E Jiao should not be cooked with the rest of this formula. After finishing the cooking process, add in the E Jiao, stir well to dissolve, and then steep the decoction for fifteen minutes, and then strain off the herbs.

Dosage for Tang or Decoction

Drink four to eight ounces of the warm strained decoction (tea), three times a day as needed.

Dosage for Powder

This formula should be taken twice daily. The powder can be taken in several different ways. Make a smoothie, by adding twenty to thirty grams of the powder to eight ounces of juice smoothie, mix well, and drink. If that is an issue we recommend adding twenty to thirty grams of the powdered herbs to 00-size capsules. For more detailed instructions, follow the step-by-step guide for preparing a smoothie or capsules discussed in Chapter Five.

Herbal Ingredients

Grams	Chinese Herb	Botanical Name	Common Name
3	Bei Mu 川贝	*Fritillariae*	Fritillaria
3	E Jiao* 阿胶	*Equus Asinus*	Ass-Hide Glue
3	Jie Geng 桔梗	*Platycodon*	Platycodon
3	Kuan Dong Hua 冬花	*Tussilago Farfara*	Coltsfoot Flowers
3	Ren Shen 人参	*Ginseng*	Ginseng
3	Sang Bai Pi 桑白皮	*Morus Alba*	Mulberry Bark
6	Wu Mei 乌梅	*Fructus Mume*	Dark Plum
3	Wu Wei Zi 五味子	*Schisandra*	Schizandra
6	Ying Su Ke 罂粟壳	*Pericarpium Papaveris*	Poppy Husk

PATENT FORMULAS

Ban Xia Wan

Pinellia Root Teapills

Therapeutic Actions

This patent formula treats tuberculosis; including by not limited to cough with phlegm, lung congestion difficulty breathing in acute bronchitis, or pneumonia.

Packaged

In bottle of two hundred pills.

Dosage
Take six pills three times daily.

Chuan Ke Ling
Cough Effective Remedy

Therapeutic Actions
This patent formula treats tuberculosis; including but not limited to labored breathing aggravated by sticky phlegm that's difficult to expectorate in bronchitis, pneumonia, lung infection and smoker's cough.

Packaged
In bottle of one hundred pills.

Dosage
Take three to four tablets, two to three times daily.

❧

ULCERATED NOSE LINING

An ulcerated nose lining is an open sore that is usually inflamed and painful inside one or both nostrils, which develop on the skin or mucous membrane that is a result of the destruction of surface nasal tissue. A common cause is snorting drugs like cocaine.

Successful Chinese medical treatment includes herbal formulas that focus on healing the tissue of the nose, which will stop the bleeding, heal the sore and relieve the pain. Discontinuing snorting drugs is something to consider, especially during treatment.

All of the herbal prescriptions that follow can be effectively used to treat ulcerated nose lining. For each prescription, I will provide its unique processing instructions and therapeutic action.

RAW HERB FORMULAS
Xie Bai San

Drain the White Powder

Therapeutic Actions

This prescription is used to treat ulcerated nose lining; it heals the tissue of the nose and stops bleeding and pain.

Preparation

Traditionally, this formula was used in the raw form to prepare a decoction; however, for those who have not developed the taste for harsh teas, we suggest the user have the ingredients ground into a fine powder by his/her herb supplier, and then store the powder in a brown or amber glass bottle with a lid.

Store it in a cool environment free of sunlight and moisture until needed — do not refrigerate.

Dosage for Tang or Decoction

Drink four ounces of the warm strained decoction (tea), three times a day as needed.

Dosage for Powder

This formula should be taken twice daily. The powder can be taken in several different ways. Make a smoothie, by adding twenty to thirty grams of the powder to eight ounces of juice smoothie, mix well, and drink. If that is an issue we recommend adding twenty to thirty grams of the powdered herbs to 00-size capsules. For more detailed instructions, follow the step-by-step guide for preparing a smoothie or capsules discussed in Chapter Five.

Herbal Ingredients

Grams	Chinese Herb	Botanical Name	Common Name
15	Di Gu Pi 地骨皮	*Lycium Barbarum*	Wolfberry
15	Sang Bai Pi 桑白皮	*Morus Alba*	Mulberry Bark
3	Zhi Gan Cao 甘草	*Glycyrrhizae*	Licorice

Contraindication

Do not use if you have a cough caused by flu or cold.

Yu Nu Jian

Jade Woman Decoction

Therapeutic Actions

This prescription is used to treat ulcerated nose lining; it relieves bleeding, primarily nosebleeds and nourishes the lining of the nose.

Preparation

Traditionally, this formula was used in the raw form to prepare a decoction; however, for those who have not developed the taste for harsh teas, we suggest the user have the ingredients ground into a fine powder by his/her herb supplier, and then store the powder in a brown or amber glass bottle with a lid. Store it in a cool environment free of sunlight and moisture until needed — do not refrigerate.

*Dosage Note

The gram weight to be used in this formula is listed with a minimum/maximum range. This prescription should be prepared by using the lower dosage and only increase dosage to achieve stronger results when needed.

Dosage for Tang or Decoction

Drink four to eight ounces of the warm strained decoction (tea), three times a day as needed.

Dosage for Powder

This formula should be taken twice daily. The powder can be taken in several different ways. Make a smoothie, by adding twenty to thirty grams of the powder to eight ounces of juice smoothie, mix well, and drink. If that is an issue we recommend adding twenty to thirty grams of the powdered herbs to 00-size capsules. For more detailed instructions, follow the step-by-step guide for preparing a smoothie or capsules discussed in Chapter Five.

Herbal Ingredients

Grams	Chinese Herb	Botanical Name	Common Name
4.5	Chuan Niu Xi 川牛膝	*Cyathula Officinalis*	Cyathula Root
6	Mai Men Dong 麦冬	*Ophiopogon*	Winter Wheat
9–15*	Shi Gao 生石膏	*Gypsum*	Gypsum
9–30*	Shu Di Huang 熟地黃	*Rehmanniae Preparata*	Rehmannia Cooked
4.5	Zhi Mu 知母	*Anemarrhena*	Anemarrhena

Contraindication

If you suffer from spleen or stomach deficiencies do not use this formula.

🍁

VOMITING

Vomiting is the involuntary expulsion of stomach contents through the mouth. It is usually preceded by nausea, pallor, sweating and a reduction in the heart rate.

Vomiting is often a result of overindulgence in food or alcohol. It can also be caused by drugs, anesthesia or disorders of the stomach or intestines. Vomiting can be caused by inflammation of organs associated with the digestive tract, such as the liver, pancreas and gallbladder.

Vomiting blood known medically as hematemesis, is a symptom of bleeding from the digestive tract that usually occurs as a result of a serious disorder of the esophagus, stomach, or duodenum. I would advise anyone who is vomiting blood to have it looked into by a medical professional to determine the exact cause.

If your stomach is churning and you're throwing up after a night of heavy drinking, or you zonked out on something else that left you with an upset stomach, one of the prescriptions that follows should help!

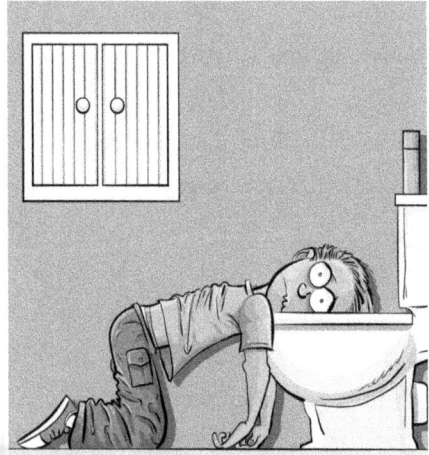

Successful Chinese herbal treatment for vomiting includes herbal formulas that heal disorders of the digestive tract and relieve the symptoms of nausea, gas, bloating, abdominal pressure, and the urge to vomit.

All of the herbal prescriptions that follow can be effectively used to treat vomiting. For each prescription, I will provide its unique processing instructions and therapeutic action.

RAW HERB FORMULAS
Bao He Wan
Preserve Harmony Decoction

Therapeutic Actions
This prescription is used to treat vomiting, including symptoms of nausea, bloating, acid regurgitation, and belching (with a foul odor).

Preparation
Traditionally, this formula was used in the raw form to prepare a decoction; however, for those who have not developed the taste for harsh teas, we suggest the user have the ingredients ground into a fine powder by his/her herb supplier, and then store the powder in a brown or amber glass

bottle with a lid. Store it in a cool environment free of sunlight and moisture until needed — do not refrigerate.

Dosage for Tang or Decoction
Drink eight ounces of the warm strained decoction (tea), as needed.

Dosage for Powder
This formula should be taken as needed. The powder can be used in several different ways. Make a smoothie, by adding twenty to thirty grams of the powder to eight ounces of juice smoothie, mix well, and drink. If that is an issue we recommend adding twenty to thirty grams of the powdered herbs to 00-size capsules. For more detailed instructions, follow the step-by-step guide for preparing a smoothie or capsules discussed in Chapter Five.

Herbal Ingredients

Grams	Chinese Herb	Botanical Name	Common Name
9	Ban Xia 半夏	*Pinellia Ternata*	Half Summer
6	Chen Pi 陳皮	*Citrus Reticulate*	Tangerine Peel
9	Fu Ling 茯苓	*Poria Cocos*	Tuckahoe
6	Lai Fu Zi 莱菔子	*Raphanus Sativus*	Radish Seed
6	Lian Qiao 连翘	*Forsythia Suspensa*	Forsythia
18	Shan Zha 山楂	*Crataegus Cuneata*	Hawthorne Fruit
6	Shen Qu 神曲	*Massa Fermentata*	Medicated Leaven

Contraindications
Do not use this formula during pregnancy. Do not eat raw food during treatment.

Note
Individuals with severe vomiting and diarrhea may experience dehydration from excessive loss of fluids. Therefore, electrolytes and fluids should be replenished.

Lian Po Yin

Coptis and Magnolia Bark Decoction

Therapeutic Actions

Used for treating excessive vomiting, with nausea, bloating, and belching.

Preparation

Traditionally, this formula was used in the raw form to prepare a decoction; however, for those who have not developed the taste for harsh teas, we suggest the user have the ingredients ground into a fine powder by his/her herb supplier, and then store the powder in a brown or amber glass bottle with a lid. Store it in a cool environment free of sunlight and moisture until needed — do not refrigerate.

Dosage for Tang or Decoction

Drink eight ounces of the warm strained decoction (tea), as needed.

Dosage for Powder

This formula should be taken as needed. The powder can be used in several different ways. Make a smoothie, by adding twenty to thirty grams of the powder to eight ounces of juice smoothie, mix well, and drink. If that is an issue we recommend adding twenty to thirty grams of the powdered herbs to 00-size capsules. For more detailed instructions, follow the step-by-step guide for preparing a smoothie or capsules discussed in Chapter Five.

Herbal Ingredients

Grams	Chinese Herb	Botanical Name	Common Name
3	Ban Xia 半夏	*Pinellia Ternata*	Half Summer
9	Dan Dou Chi 淡豆豉	*Sojae Preparatum*	Soybean
6	Hou Po 厚朴	*Magnolia Officinalis*	Magnolia Bark
3	Huang Lian 黃連	*Coptis*	Coptis Root
60	Lu Gen 芦根	*Phragmitis*	Reed Rhizome
3	Shi Chang Pu 石菖蒲	*Acori*	Acorus
9	Zhi Zi 栀子	*Gardenia*	Gardenia

Note

Individuals with severe vomiting and diarrhea may experience dehydration from excessive loss of fluids. Therefore, electrolytes and fluids should be replenished.

🍁

WITHDRAWAL

With breathless anticipation the rubber bulb is squeezed ever so gently as the heroin slowly exits the syringe and silently enters the bloodstream. Soon a warm flush spreads over the skin as perspiration rises to the surface allowing tension to escape through the open pores. As the arms and legs become increasingly heavy and relaxed, the circadian rhythm gradually deaccelerates winding down to slow motion as the user peacefully departs from reality and little by little, enters the land of nod...

Even though withdrawal from drugs and alcohol both have their own unique challenges, many of the mental and physical symptoms experienced by someone, who regularly gets high and suddenly stops, are quite similar. Regardless of which substance you're withdrawing from, when it reaches this point, long-term users must come to terms with the fact that for the next four to seven days—especially the first two or three when the symptoms are most intense—saying that you're going to be feeling like shit might be an understatement!

Withdrawal from opiates like heroin or morphine usually starts eight to twelve hours after the last hit and can last for five to ten days. At first a craving for the drug is the most prominent symptom, soon it is accompanied by sweating, fever, chills and runny eyes and nose, muscle spasms and deep bone pain. Some people withdrawing from opiates describe it as feeling like the worst flu they ever experienced. As withdrawal progresses, other symptoms appear such as diarrhea, vomiting, abdominal cramps, dilated pupils, loss of appetite, the cold sweats or goosebumps (which is where the term cold turkey came from), irritability, tremors, weakness, depression, and occasionally suicidal thoughts.

Alcohol withdrawal symptoms usually start six to eight hours after the last drink. Common symptoms include the shakes (trembling of the hands and tongue), confusion, sweating, rapid heart-rate, nausea, dilated pupils, involuntary movement of the eyelids, irritability, anxiety, diarrhea, disturbed sleep (insomnia or nightmares), and sometimes there are stomach cramps and vomiting. More severe symptoms include seizures and hallucinations.

Other drugs like codeine and some of the prescription analgesics cause withdrawal symptoms similar to those produced by heroin or morphine, but when they are used in smaller doses; symptoms can be less intense and may develop more slowly. Withdrawal from speed (amphetamines) and cocaine includes symptoms such as dizziness and extreme fatigue, agitation, anxiety, depression and occasionally suicidal tendencies. Normally, the physical withdrawal symptoms from cocaine do not have the same intensity as withdrawal from opiates. Typically, barbiturate (tranquilizers) withdrawal begins twelve to twenty-four hours after the last dose and is very similar to alcohol withdrawal. Symptoms of withdrawal from drugs like ecstasy include panic attacks, anxiety, paranoia, delusions, irritability and insomnia.

When drinking or drug use is discontinued and alcohol/drugs leave the body of the user—who has been getting high on a regular basis for a long period of time — any of the following symptoms can occur. Chinese herbal formulas can be successfully used to treat many of these symptoms: abdominal pain, accelerated heartrate, agitation, alcoholic convulsions, anxiety, body aches, chills, delirium tremens, diarrhea, disorientation, epileptic seizures, fear, fever, hallucinations, headache, insomnia, labored breathing, muscle ache, nausea, perspiration, profuse sweating, rapid pulse, restlessness, runny nose, seizures, shaking, tremors, vomiting, and watery eyes. The herbal formulas in this category can be used to reduce some of the symptoms of withdrawal. However, I feel that it's important to remind the reader that withdrawal symptoms that are a result of long-term addiction can be severe and in some cases life-threatening. Therefore, you may want to consider seeking professional Western medical help.

RAW HERB FORMULAS
Wu Zhu Yu Tang
Evodia Decoction

Therapeutic Actions
This prescription is used to treat withdrawal from both inhalation and injection drugs; it relieves vomiting, feeling of fullness, distention of chest and stomach, epigastric pain, belching, acid regurgitation, headache, dry heaves, diarrhea, cold hands and feet, severe shaking or fidgeting, irritability, fatigue, poor appetite, and vomiting of clear fluids.

Preparation
Traditionally, this formula was used in the raw form to prepare a decoction; however, for those who have not developed the taste for harsh teas, we suggest the user have the ingredients ground into a fine powder by his/her herb supplier, and then store the powder in a brown or amber glass bottle with a lid. Store it in a cool environment free of sunlight and moisture until needed — do not refrigerate.

*Preparation Note
The herb Sheng Jiang or fresh ginger should not be cooked for longer than five minutes. Do not add it to the herbs being cooked until the last five minutes of preparation time.

*Dosage Note

The gram weight to be used in this formula is listed with a minimum/maximum range. This prescription should be prepared by using the lower dosage and only increase dosage to achieve stronger results when needed.

Dosage for Tang or Decoction

Drink four ounces of the warm strained decoction (tea), three times daily, as needed.

Dosage for Powder

This formula should be taken as needed. The powder can be used in several different ways. Make a smoothie, by adding twenty to thirty grams of the powder to eight ounces of juice smoothie, mix well, and drink. If that is an issue we recommend adding twenty to thirty grams of the powdered herbs to 00-size capsules. For more detailed instructions, follow the step-by-step guide for preparing a smoothie or capsules discussed in Chapter Five.

Herbal Ingredients

Grams	Chinese Herb	Botanical Name	Common Name
9	Bai Zhu 白朮	*Atractylodes*	Atractylodes
4 Pieces	Da Zao 大棗	*Ziziphus Jujuba*	Jujube
15	Fu Ling 茯苓	*Poria Cocos*	Tuckahoe
6	Ren Shen 人参	*Ginseng*	Ginseng
18	Sheng Jiang* 生姜	*Zingiber Officinale*	Ginger Sliced
3-9*	Wu Zhu Yu* 吳茱萸	*Evodia*	Evodia

Ge Hua Jie Cheng San

Pueraria Flower Powder for Detoxification and Awakening

Therapeutic Actions

This prescription is used to relieve the symptoms of an alcohol hangover; it will stop vomiting, relieve headache, dizziness, chest distention, lack of appetite and fatigue. Use for quick recovery from alcohol intoxication, this formula is famous for its ability to quickly restore sobriety.

Preparation

Traditionally, this formula was used in the raw form to prepare a decoction; however, for those who have not developed the taste for harsh teas, we suggest the user have the ingredients ground into a fine powder by his/her herb supplier, and then store the powder in a brown or amber glass bottle with a lid. Store it in a cool environment free of sunlight and moisture until needed — do not refrigerate.

Dosage for Tang or Decoction

Make a tea by adding nine grams of the powder to eight ounces of boiling water allow it to steep for fifteen minutes and drink. Do this three times during the day as needed.

Dosage for Powder

This formula should be taken three times during the day as needed. The powder can be used in several different ways.

Make a smoothie, by adding twenty to thirty grams of the powder to eight ounces of juice smoothie, mix well, and drink. If that is an issue we recommend adding twenty to thirty grams of the powdered herbs to 00-size capsules. For more detailed instructions, follow the step-by-step guide for preparing a smoothie or capsules discussed in Chapter Five.

Herbal Ingredients

Grams	Chinese Herb	Botanical Name	Common Name
15	Bai Dou Kou 白豆蔻	*Amomim*	Cardamom
6	Bai Zhu 白朮	*Atractylodes*	Atractylodes
4.5	Chen Pi 陳皮	*Citrus Reticulate*	Tangerine Peel
4.5	Fu Ling 茯苓	*Poria Cocos*	Tuckahoe
6	Gan Jiang 乾薑	*Zingiber*	Ginger Dried
15	Ge Hua 葛花	*Flos Puerariae*	Kudzu
0.9	Lian Fang 蓮房	*Nelumbo*	Lotus Leaf
1.5	Mu Xiang 木香	*Aucklandiae*	Costus
1.5	Qing Pi 青皮	*Citrus Reticulata*	Tangerine Peel
4.5	Ren Shen 人參	*Ginseng*	Ginseng
15	Sha Ren 砂仁	*Amomum*	Amomum
6	Shen Qu 神曲	*Massa*	Leaven
6	Ze Xie 澤瀉	*Alisma Orientalis*	Water Plantain
4.5	Zhu Ling 豬苓	*Polyporus*	Polyporus

PATENT HERB FORMULA
Chai Hu Long Gu Mu Li Wan

Bupleurum, Dragon Bone, and Oyster Shell Pills

Therapeutic Actions

This patent formula is used to treat withdrawal; it relieves vomiting, feeling of fullness, distention of chest and stomach, epigastric pain, belching, acid regurgitation, headache, dry heaves, diarrhea, cold hands and feet, severe shaking or fidgeting, irritability, fatigue, poor appetite, and vomiting of clear fluids.

Caution

Do not use during pregnancy.

Packaged

In bottle of two hundred pills.

Dosage

Take eight pills, three times per day. Dosage can be increase to twelve pills, if needed.

Commentary

You may have noticed that the two formulas used for treating withdrawal pretty much do the same thing (I'm referring to *Wu Zhu Yu Tang* vs. *Chai Hu Long Gu Mu Li Wan*). The difference in the two prescriptions, other than the fact that the raw herb formula requires preparation, and the other does not, is their speed of action. The decision about which formula to use probably seems like a no-brainer, but before you rush to a decision that's based entirely on convenience and minimal effort, you owe it to yourself to give some thought to what I'm about to say: 1) When raw herbs are decocted or made into tea, they can be sipped slowly at a pace that's comfortable for the patient, as opposed to gulping down the prescribed dosage of pills in one fell swoop. 2) When herbal tea is drunk warm it can help reduce the chills as well as warm cold hands and feet which are common symptoms of withdrawal, and 3) Not only is taking medicine in pill form a more impersonal way of administering medicine, because of the time that's needed for pills to be broken down in the stomach and absorbed and assimilated by the body, normally it takes longer for its therapeutic effects to be felt.

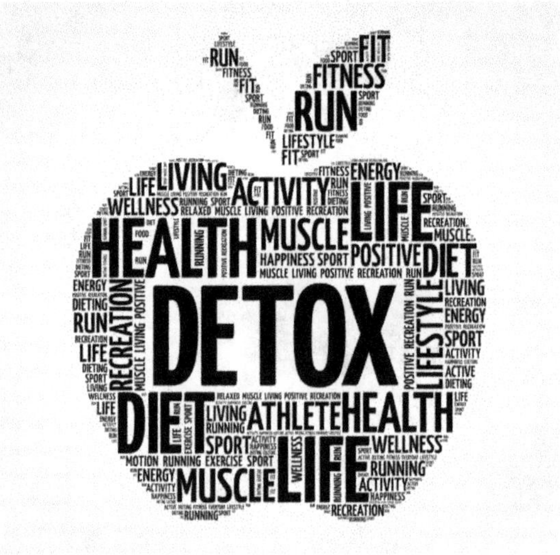

RUN
FIT
FITNESS
RUN
LIFESTYLE
LIVING
ACTIVITY
ENERGY
LIFE
WELLNESS
HEALTH
MUSCLE
HAPPINESS SPORT
POSITIVE
DIET
DETOX
RECREATION
LIFESTYLE
LIVING
ENERGY
SPORT
RUN
LIFE
DIET
LIVING
ATHLETE
HEALTH
SPORT
WELLNESS
MOTION RUNNING EXERCISE SPORT
MUSCLE
LIFE
RUNNING
ACTIVITY
RECREATION

CHAPTER FOUR

Detox and Internal Cleansing

Methods and Formulas

This chapter was written for people who want to breathe new life into bodies that suffer from the lingering effects of alcohol and drug use. It should be of particular interest to those for whom raves, rock concerts, and weekends at the club are a thing of the past, who might be considering detox as a follow-up therapy after withdrawal, as part of recovery after an illness, or by someone who has simply reached a point in his/her life and want to reverse some of the damage caused by too much partying, fast food and a few other indiscretions that are typically part of our "coming of age."

I will discuss internal cleansing and provide formulas that eliminate residual toxins from the body, along with some prescriptions for what Chinese Herbology calls Longevity Tonics; these are effective herbal formulas that rejuvenate and strengthen the body.

Both health regimens (internal cleansing and longevity tonics) are highly recommended for anyone interested in improving his/her overall health, especially those with a history of alcohol or drug use. Although generally speaking every organ in our body is affected by what we put in it, when it comes to alcohol and drugs, the organs that filter toxins from the blood, namely the liver and kidneys, are a particular concern.

Even though one would be hard pressed to find a health-conscious person who would argue against organ cleansing, there are varying opinions about the impact of the adjunctive therapy on health.

Some hard-core naturopaths and members of the holistic health community strongly recommend regular (annual or semi-annual) cleansing of the body's blood purifying apparatus (primarily the liver and kidneys) as part of a health maintenance strategy. The list of ailments that benefit from organ cleansing according to these health enthusiasts include everything from overweight/obesity, nausea or other chronic digestive problems, hepatitis, gallstones, diabetes or hypoglycemia, chronic fatigue, thyroid condition, food chemical and environmental allergies, high cholesterol, and fibromyalgia. Secondary benefits include increased energy, improved appearance of the skin, clearer eyes, more mental alertness, better digestion and elimination, and increased metabolism.

In fairness I should mention there are also naturalists and health enthusiasts who agree that detoxification does have some merits, but believe its benefits are sometime over-rated. My personal opinion is for anyone who has a history–of substance abuse–whether alcohol, drugs or fast food--organ cleansing is worth considering.

However, before I get into the details of internal cleansing and some of the formulas that are used to remove toxic buildup, I'd like to take a moment to describe each organ's anatomical location, and give a brief explanation about what it does.

The Liver

The largest of the five internal organs, the liver occupies the upper right-hand portion of the abdominal cavity. Aided by the kidneys, one of the functions of the liver is to filter the blood of toxic by-products from food additives and pesticides as well as environmental pollutants such as heavy metals, and potentially harmful residual toxins from things like drugs and alcohol. These health-endangering substances, that would otherwise accumulate in the bloodstream, are absorbed by the liver, made water-soluble by altering their chemical structure, and excreted in the bile. Over the years the residue from this waste material builds up and it can undermine the organs ability to function efficiently.

The Kidneys

The kidneys assist the liver in filtering the blood by excreting waste products in fluid/liquids and excess water in the form of urine. An important component of the body's filtration system, the kidneys are located in the lower abdomen around the waistline, one underneath the liver on the right and the other underneath the spleen on the left. Separate but equal, the kidneys and liver work in tandem. Even though there's evidence that kidney disease occurs more often in people who use drugs and heavy drinkers are more likely to suffer from diseases affecting the liver, it really doesn't matter which one was your preferred method for getting high—I can't overstate the importance of detoxifying both the kidneys and the liver in order to completely flush out the system.

If you have any lingering doubts about the benefits of organ cleansing, let me assure you that every person I have known who has done a complete twenty-one-day detoxification says the same thing, and I quote: "You know I don't know exactly how to describe it, but overall I just feel better."

Organ Cleanse

Most people in reasonably good health can follow these guidelines for detox. However, if you have any health issues such as hypertension, cancer, diabetes, congestive heart failure, etc., then I suggest that you check with a health care professional (your doctor) before starting organ cleansing to make certain that the therapy does not pose any health risks, and the herbal formulas do not conflict with any prescriptions.

Each organ should be detoxed separately and the process takes seven to ten days. Whether you do the kidneys first or the liver is your choice, any order is acceptable.

The complete detox, cleansing both the liver and kidneys takes two to three weeks (three weeks being optimal), and is highly recommended for anyone who is currently using or has a history of using alcohol, drugs, anabolic steroids, birth control pills, or hormone replacement therapy. Trust me you'll be glad you did!

How to Perform a Kidney Cleanse

1. Drink adequate amounts of water (eight cups to two liters) distilled, filtered or spring water daily. Running a lot of water through the system for a couple of weeks will flush out waste and improve circulation to the organ.
2. Follow a low-protein diet. Avoid animal protein, meat, dairy products, poultry, seafood, chocolate, and other caffeinated products to eliminate further buildup of calcium oxalate and uric acid. Eat fresh fruit and organic vegetables and legumes and seeds, cranberry juice, and algae products, such as spirulina, chlorella—are all good. Eating melons and vegetables containing a high percentage of water that encourage

urination like watermelon, celery, beansprouts and cucumbers will all to help flush the kidneys and the bladder.

3. Drink eight to twelve ounces of the detox formula daily.

How to Perform a Liver Cleanse

1. To cleanse the liver avoid eating animal products and maintain a diet consisting of high-fiber fruits, vegetables, seeds, nuts and legumes. Drink plenty of water (at least six to twelve cups of filtered or spring water daily). Avoid saturated fats, refined sugar, and alcohol. Vegetable and fruit juices are highly recommended, as well as apples, beets, broccoli, brown rice, Brussel sprouts, cabbage, carrots, dandelion, oat bran, spinach, tomatoes, walnuts, caraway seeds, artichokes, asparagus and garlic.

2. Drink eight to twelve ounces of detox formula daily.

The most important steps required to detox both the liver and kidneys are an increased intake of raw natural foods, especially fruits and vegetables, and taking in plenty of liquids, in the form of water, vegetable and fruit juices. Some of the best options for juices are: beets, kale, parsley, blueberries, kiwi, and cranberries, which can be consumed separately or blended together into a juice cocktail.

Using Herbal Tonics to Invigorate and Strengthen after an Organ Detox

Traditional Chinese medicine considers the vital energy also known as Chi, and the blood which it refers to as the vital fluid, the two most important elements in human physiology. It is a fundamental belief of the ancient medicine that abundant health and optimal physical fitness are profoundly influenced by the condition of these two essential physiological components.

According to the five-thousand-year-old medical system the way to enhance the quality of these two vital elements is by nourishing, supplementing, and enriching them with herbal tonics. Since its creation and throughout the history of Chinese herbal medicine, volumes have been written about the benefits of using herbal nutriments to invigorate and strengthen the body. This proven ability of specific herbal prescriptions to strengthen and invigorate is the primary reason that Chinese medicine frequently prescribes Chi tonics to restore the strength and vitality of patients following illness.

Not only is herbal medicine an important part of patient recovery, Chi tonics are also frequently used for improving the health of people who are in relatively good health — whose goal is simply to increase their energy, achieve maximal wellness, and live a long healthy life.

Using Chinese herbal tonics to promote life extension and improve one's health is a Taoist tradition that dates back thousands of years. The herbal life-style of the Taoist nature-based religious sect, and their use of herbs to nourish and invigorate the blood and Chi in what they refer to as "Longevity Formulas," has been written about extensively in Taoist literature. Followers of the quasi-mystical religion are well-known for their radiant health and the fact that it's not uncommon for them to live healthy vibrant lives well into advanced age. On the pages that follow you will find some of the most famous Taoist Longevity Formulas.

DETOX FORMULA
Triple Leaf Detox Tea
Cleansing and Revitalizing Tea

Therapeutic Actions
This patent formula is used to detox both the liver and kidneys; it contains purifying herbs that support healthy functioning of the liver, kidneys, lungs and blood, and is used to cleanse the body of toxins.

Packaged
In box of twenty teabags.

Dosage
Drink eight to twelve ounces of tea daily for seven to ten days (per organ to be cleansed) and eat the diet previously discussed.

LONGEVITY FORMULAS

Yan Nian Yi Shou

Live 100 Years Longevity Tonic

Therapeutic Actions

This powerful tonic combines fifteen ingredients that are renowned in the Chinese and Taoist healthy systems for their ability to enhance the functioning of the body's vital organs (especially the kidneys, liver, heart, lungs and spleen). These herbs will strengthen the functioning of the immune system (the Wei Chi), delaying the physical debilitation that accompanies the aging process.

Preparation

Traditionally, this formula was used in the raw form to prepare a decoction; however, for those who have not developed the taste for harsh teas, we suggest the user have the ingredients ground into a fine powder by his/her herb supplier, and then store the powder in a brown or amber glass bottle with a lid. Store it in a cool environment free of sunlight and moisture until needed — do not refrigerate.

Dosage for Tang or Decoction

Make a tea by adding nine grams of the powder to eight ounces of boiling water allow it to steep for fifteen minutes and drink. Do this three times during the day.

Dosage for Powder

This formula should be taken two to three times daily. The powder can be used in several different ways. Make a smoothie, by adding twenty to thirty grams of the powder to eight ounces of juice smoothie, mix well, and drink. If that is an issue we recommend adding twenty to thirty grams of the powdered herbs to 00-size capsules. For more detailed instructions, follow the step-by-step guide for preparing a smoothie or capsules discussed in Chapter Five.

Herbal Ingredients

Grams	Chinese Herb	Botanical Name	Common Name
12	Bai Zhu 白朮	*Atractylodes*	Atractylodes
25	Bing Tang 冰糖	*Raw Sugar*	Sugar
22	Da Zao 大棗	*Ziziphus Jujuba*	Jujube
30	Dang Shen 党参	*Codonoposis*	Codonopsis
18	Fang Feng 防風	*Ledebouriellae*	Siler
18	Fu Shen 茯神	*Poriae*	Hoelen Center
12	Gou Qi Zi 枸杞子	*Lycii Fructus*	Wolfberry
24	Huang Qi 黃芪	*Astragalus*	Milkvetch Root
12	Mai Men Dong 麦冬	*Ophiopogon*	Winter Wheat
18	Qiang Huo 羌活	*Notopterygum*	Notopteygium
10	Rou Gui 肉桂	*Cinnamomum*	Cinnamon
20	Shan Zhu Yu 山茱萸	*Corni Fructus*	Dogwood Fruit
18	Sheng Di Huang 生地黃	*Rehmanniae*	Rehmannia
18	Shu Di Huang 熟地黃	*Rehmanniae Preparata*	Rehmannia Cooked
18	Wu Wei Zi 五味子	*Schisandra*	Schizandra

Contraindications

Caution is recommended when using this formula for women who are pregnant, and when breast feeding an infant.

Si Jun Zi Tang

Four-Gentlemen Decoction

Therapeutic Actions

This is the most frequently used blood tonic in traditional Chinese medicine; it was first mentioned in Shen Nong's classic Ben Cao Jing, thousands of years ago. The formula's widespread use is prompted by traditional Chinese medicine's assertion, which by nourishing and enriching the blood, anemia and associated fatigue is avoided. By regulating the blood, all of the vital organs benefit, and by circulating the blood, flexibility and movement of the joints is improved.

Preparation

Traditionally, this formula was used in the raw form to prepare a decoction; however, for those who have not developed the taste for harsh teas, we suggest the user have the ingredients ground into a fine powder by his/her herb supplier, and then store the powder in a brown or amber glass bottle with a lid. Store it in a cool environment free of sunlight and moisture until needed — do not refrigerate.

Dosage for Tang or Decoction

Make a tea by adding nine grams of the powder to eight ounces of boiling water allow it to steep for fifteen minutes and drink. Do this three times during the day.

Dosage for Powder

This formula should be taken two to three times daily. The powder can be used in several different ways. Make a smoothie, by adding twenty to thirty grams of the powder to eight ounces of juice smoothie, mix well, and drink. If that is an issue we recommend adding twenty to thirty grams of the powdered herbs to 00-size capsules. For more detailed instructions, follow the step-by-step guide for preparing a smoothie or capsules discussed in Chapter Five.

Herbal Ingredients

Grams	Chinese Herb	Botanical Name	Common Name
9	Bai Zhu 白术	Atractylodes	Atractylodes
9	Fu Ling 茯苓	Poria Cocos	Tuckahoe
9	Ren Shen 人参	Ginseng	Ginseng
9	Zhi Gan Cao 甘草	Glycyrrhizae	Licorice

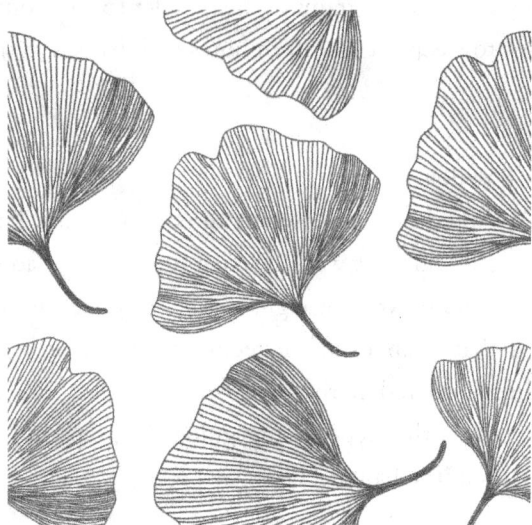

CHAPTER FIVE

Preparing Herbal Pharmaceuticals

B efore we get into the different ways that an herbal formula can be prepared, there are three things that need to be taken into consideration:

The quality of the herbs...

The key to preparing potent pharmaceuticals is the quality of the herbs that are used. Most formulas sold commercially are made with herbs of inferior quality, consequently, the potency and effectiveness of the resulting formula is less than those prepared with high quality ingredients. Therefore, I suggest that you prepare the herbal formula, using high-quality herbs. Generally speaking, higher quality herbs are packaged in sealed containers and are slightly more expensive than herbs of inferior quality that are displayed loose in boxes and bins.

The herbs freshness...

Of equal importance is the freshness of the herbs that are used. When herbs are used that are past their prime, the result is a less potent formula. Moistness, pliability, and aroma, are usually good indicators of an herb's freshness. Herbs devoid of fragrance, that are dry brittle, and in fragments or pieces, are usually past their prime.

How the formulas are stored...

There are those who claim that storing an herbal prescription in plastic bottles is acceptable; well, let me stress to you that nothing could be further from the truth. Using glass containers will prevent the chemical changes that plastic will cause, which are known to undermine the efficacy of the medicinal substances. Also avoid storing the container in sunlight; an environment that is neither hot nor cold is preferred. I also recommend that you use amber glass containers rather than plain glass to avoid the penetration of light.

What follows are the processing instructions and methods of preparation. Each method of preparation is listed by its English and Chinese designation followed by step-by-step instructions.

Step-by-Step Processing Instructions for
Herbal Formulas
Decoction | *Tang*
Pills or Capsules | *Wan or Pian*
Smoothie | *Bing Sha*

♣

How to Prepare a Decoction
Tang

There is no question that decoction or tang—the Chinese translation for soup—is the most popular method of using Chinese herbal medicine. It is the method of choice for several important reasons. The main reason being that medicinal ingredients prepared in this fashion are absorbed and assimilated by the body more quickly, which expedites healing. I should also mention that it is a viable method of preparation for anyone who has an aversion to alcohol and can't drink an herbal formula that's been prepared into a Jiu (medicinal wine). Below are step-by-step instructions on how to prepare a tang or herbal decoction.

What is a decoction?
A traditional Chinese medicine decoction is the cooking process by which raw herbs are boiled in water and the resulting liquid (or tea) is drunk. It is very important to follow each step in the process correctly to achieve the desired effects.

How does it taste?
Perhaps I should mention that (to the uninitiated) the flavor of some herbal decoctions can definitely be less than tasty, which has prompted me to come up with a solution to that problem… two different methods of preparation. For the purist, we have the traditional method that is often beyond the taste tolerance level of the average individual, and a revised or

diluted version that is much more palatable.

Can't I just add some sugar to it?

Some do. I prefer to keep a bowl of yellow raisins handy; if I run into a particularly nasty brew, I chew a few raisins, which will clear the pallet of any unpleasant flavor.

What materials are needed?

- decocting pot with a lid
- raw herb ingredients
- water
- glass container for storage
- large strainer

Instructions for the "traditional" method of decocting (a tang):

1. Place the herbs in the pot, add enough cold water to cover the herbs by two inches, and soak the herbs in the cold water for thirty to sixty minutes; this will aid in the extraction process.

2. After the soaking process is completed, put the pot on the stove, turn the flame to high, and bring the water to a rolling boil. Stir and turn the heat down to a low simmer; cover the pot and simmer for thirty minutes.

3. Turn off the heat, remove the pot to a cool burner, and leave the decoction in the covered pot to steep for another thirty minutes.

4. Strain the herbs from the fluid; pour the tea into a glass container. You should have about six to eight ounces of condensed tea; this is considered one dose.

5. Allow the tea to cool to room temperature and drink.

6. Repeating the above process, the herbs can be cooked a second time. Normally it is recommended that a formula be taken twice daily (in the morning and evening). It is not advisable to cook the herbs more than two times (as the herbs will have lost their effectiveness).

Note

I should mention that the traditional method of preparation is not exactly cost-effective. Because the herbs are cooked in such a condensed fashion yielding only one to two doses, this does not compare favorably with the revised method (that follows) which produces a much larger yield, which lasts ten to fifteen days and under normal circumstances, is equally as effective.

Instructions for the "revised" method of decocting (a tang):

1. Place the herbs in the pot, add one gallon of cold water to the herbs, and soak the herbs in the cold water for thirty to sixty minutes; this will aid in the extraction process.

2. After the soaking process is completed, put the pot on the stove, turn the flame to high, and bring the water to a rolling boil. Stir and turn the heat down to a low simmer; cover the pot and simmer for thirty minutes.

3. Turn off the heat, remove the pot to a cool burner, and leave the decoction in the covered pot to steep for another thirty minutes.

4. Strain the herbs from the fluid, allow the tea to cool down, then pour four to eight ounces of the tea into a cup (for the first dose), and pour the remaining tea into a glass container that can hold at least one half-gallon. Once the tea is cool enough, cover with a tight lid, and store the tang in the refrigerator. It should last about two weeks.

5. Subsequent doses are either warmed on the stove or allowed to naturally come to room temperature before consumption.

🍁

How to Prepare Pills or Capsules
Wan

Herbs prepared in pill form—what is known as wan in Chinese—is the third most popular method of preparation after decoction and medicinal wine. In recent years a large number of herb users have opted to use capsules because of the convenience of storing them, and the fact that when herbs are encapsulated, the user can avoid the bitter taste that is characteristic of some herbs and formulas. Although this is a nontraditional method, the use of capsules rather than pills does not compromise the effectiveness of herbs prepared in this manner; however, it does slow down the absorption rate. By how much? Actually each body is different and much depends on whether or not the stomach is empty.

Many who find the whole decocting process simply too much of a bother, can prepare their raw herb formula into pills or capsules. On the following pages are step-by-step instructions for preparing pills or capsules.

How are pills made?

The herbs in your raw herb formula must be ground down into a fine powder (by the herb supplier or you can use the kitchen blender). If you're doing this at home in your blender, don't dump all the herbs into the blender at once, first cut the bigger sticks and branches into smaller pieces and blend those, and as they are a harder substance expect this to take a few minutes, then add in the small leaves, seeds, and flowers (which are much softer and will blend quicker). The resulting powder should be mixed with a viscous or sticky medium, rolled in the palm of your hand and shaped into a pill form and allowed to dry. The dried pills can be stored in the refrigerator for several weeks. Typical dosage is one to three pills two times daily, but check the specific formula for exact dosage instructions.

How are capsules made?

It may seem complicated but it isn't; the herbs must first be ground down into a fine powder (by the herb supplier or you can use the kitchen blender). You'll need 00-sized gelatin capsules which can be purchased from an online provider or a local drug store. Simply pour the powdered herbs into the 00-sized capsules. The capsules can be stored indefinitely in a tightly sealed glass container (do not store in the refrigerator). Typical dosage is one to three pills two times daily, but check the specific formula for exact dosage instructions.

Will it be as effective as a decocted tea?

Yes, as long as you follow each step in the process correctly, using raw herbs of the highest quality to achieve the desired effects.

Do I chew the pill or swallow it with water?

Some do chew the pills, because the typical handmade pills are bigger than a 00-sized capsule, which makes them almost impossible to swallow. I get around that issue by cutting mine in half or into quarters, which makes them easier to swallow. This is probably why most people just make their own capsules; 00-sized caps are certainly easier to swallow.

What about special preparation instructions?

Many herbal formulas that are made into pills or capsules mention dipping an herb first in vinegar or another substance. To do this, just put the herb into cider or distilled vinegar as many times as instructed. Allow the herbs to completely dry before grinding it in your blender.

Is this still considered a "traditional" method of preparing an herbal formula?

Yes, traditionally many herbal formulas were prepared as pills; however, in modern times the capsule method has become the preferred method; and both can be used without any fear of compromising the effectiveness of the formula.

How to Make Pills

What materials are needed to make pills?

- large ceramic bowl (to hold at least two quarts)
- raw herb ingredients - powdered
- honey

- gallon-size glass container with a lid, for storage
- large sifter
- large platter or aluminum foil

Step-by-step instructions for making pills

1. Sift the powdered herbs into the large ceramic bowl to separate fine from coarse particles. Toss out any coarse particles that did not powder well.
2. Once the finely-powdered herb is in the bowl, pour in a viscous or sticky medium like honey. Not too much, the object here is to mix in a little honey and then stir the mixture checking to see if the consistency is correct. The resulting mix should be dry enough to be molded into pills, yet not so dry it crumbles and won't stick together.
3. Take a small amount of the mixture into the palm of your hand and roll it into the shape of a small bean or pea. Don't make them any larger because it will be too large to swallow easily.
4. Continue rolling the mixture into small pills and place those beans on a non-stick surface like a large sheet of aluminum foil, a cookie sheet, or a serving platter.
5. Allow the pills to dry. This process could take a few days.
6. Be sure to allow the pills as much time as they need to dry, otherwise your pills will stick together when they are stored.
7. Place the dried pills into a large glass jar with a lid and close the lid.
8. Refrigerate the jar; it should stay fresh for several weeks.

How to Make Capsules

What materials are needed to make capsules?

- three large ceramic bowls (each should hold at least two quarts)
- raw herb ingredients – powdered
- 00-sized gelatin capsules
- quart-sized glass container with a lid, for storage
- large sifter

- gallon-sized plastic baggies
- paper towel

Step-by-step instructions for making capsules

1. Cover the work area with paper towel, as this process can get dusty.
2. Put about one hundred of the 00-sized capsules into a large ceramic bowl.
3. Sift the powdered herbs into another large ceramic bowl, to separate fine from coarse particles. Toss out any coarse particles that did not powder well.
4. Once the finely-powdered herb is in the bowl, you can either make the capsules in that bowl or pour the powder into a large plastic baggie. Some find working in a plastic baggie keeps the herb-dust to a minimum.
5. Open the 00-sized capsules and fill the larger half with powder then close the two halves.
6. Put the filled capsule into a large ceramic bowl.
7. Store the filled capsules in a larger glass container with a lid, or in a large baggie.
8. Do not store the caps in the refrigerator; keep the container on a dry and dark (no sunlight) shelf.
9. The capsules can be stored for a fairly long period of time and remain usable.

❧

How to Prepare an Herbal Smoothie
Bing Sha

Using Chinese herbs to make a Smoothie

Although the decoction/medicinal wine process are commonly used when preparing herbal tonics, raw herb formulas can easily be made into a smoothie. Many who find the whole decocting and aging process simply too much of a bother, can prepare their raw herb formula into a smoothie. And, although assimilation is somewhat slower you can still be assured the formula will be just as effective as if it were prepared as a decoction or medicinal wine. What follows are step-by-step instructions on how to prepare a smoothie.

How is the smoothie made?

The Chinese herbs in your raw herb formula must be ground down into a fine powder (by your herbalist or you can use a kitchen blender or coffee grinder). If you're powdering the herbs at home, don't dump all the herbs into the blender at once, first cut the bigger sticks and branches into smaller pieces and blend those, and as they are a harder substance expect this to take a few minutes, then add in the small leaves, seeds, and flowers (which are much softer and will blend quicker). The resulting powder should be mixed with fruit, juice and sweetener and blended to prepare a smoothie. Complete instructions on how to prepare a smoothie follow. Typical dosage is to drink four to eight ounces of the smoothie daily but check the specific guidelines (for the herbal prescription) for exact dosage.

Will it be as effective as a decocted tea?

Yes, as long as you follow each step in the process correctly, use raw herbs that you are certain are of the highest quality and you will achieve the desired effects.

Step-By-Step Instructions in Making a Smoothie

Indeed, smoothies can be a nutritious and convenient meal replacement or refreshing way to consume Chinese herbal prescriptions. They're very easy to make, as well. Just a few basic ingredients blended together will render you a delicious smoothie in no time. To make a smoothie simply:

- Take out your blender or food processor.
- Start with the fruit combination of your choice. Fresh or frozen fruit

will make up the base of your smoothie; however, you can make a delicious smoothie with reconstituted dried fruit. You can focus on one fruit, or add several. Here are some options to consider: bananas, apples, avocados, kiwis, peaches, strawberries, blueberries, raspberries, mangoes, pomegranates, oranges, watermelon, pineapple, etc. If you're looking for a good starter combination, try strawberry-banana-orange.

■ Add liquid. The other main part of your smoothie is the liquid you choose to add to it. Here are some possibilities: milk, soy milk, Greek yogurt, nut milk (such as almond or coconut), fruit juice or concentrate ice cream, sherbet or frozen yogurt, or sparkling water.

■ Add powdered Chinese herb; refer to the dosage amount described on the herbal prescription.

■ Add a sweetener (to taste) such as: sugar, ripe bananas, honey, or agave nectar.

■ Add ice cubes (optional). Once everything's in the blender, put some ice cubes on top. For a single-serving smoothie, three or four should be plenty.

■ Put the lid on the blender, and turn it on medium. Then turn on puree for about one minute.

■ Turn off the blender and drink.

🍁

Contents

RESOURCES AND INDEXES

Appendix Section

Appendix Section I

What to Do in a First Aid and Emergency

- Call 911 if the person has collapsed and/or stopped breathing
- What you can do to help:
  - If the person has passed out from drugs or drinking too much alcohol, turn him/her on their side to prevent choking on vomit!
  - Begin CPR, if the person has stopped breathing or him/her breathing is dangerously weak.
  - Call Poison Control at 800-222-1222. Poison control experts will advise you how to proceed, ask if you should:
  - Attempt to make the person vomit
  - Give him/her anything to eat or drink
  - (if you have any) activated charcoal, can it be given by mouth to absorb the drug
  - Provide information or a sample of the drug the person is known to have taken to the emergency medical team.
  - Follow–up. If the person is taken to a hospital ER there is a chance that his/her stomach may need to be pumped.

Appendix Section II

Glossary of Chinese and Western Medical Terms

Acupuncture – stimulation of specific acupoints along the skin and body.

AIDS / HIV – Acquired immune deficiency syndrome or acquired immunodeficiency syndrome is caused by the virus HIV (Human Immunodeficiency Virus). The illness alters the immune system, causing vulnerability to infections and diseases.

Alcohol Poisoning – Alcohol poisoning is a serious and sometimes deadly consequence of drinking large amounts of alcohol in a short period of time.

Alkyl Nitrite – a group of chemical compounds based upon the molecular structure R-ONO. Formally they are alkyl esters of nitrous acid.

Alprazolam – aka Xanax; alprazolam is used to treat anxiety disorders, panic disorders, and anxiety.

Alzheimer's Disease – an irreversible, progressive brain disorder that slowly destroys memory and thinking skills, and eventually the ability to carry out the simplest tasks.

Amobarbital (Amytal) – a drug that is a barbiturate derivative. It has sedative-hypnotic properties.

Amphetamine – dextroamphetamine and methamphetamine, are all amphetamines. Their chemical properties and actions are so similar that even experienced users have difficulty knowing which drug they have taken.

An Intimate History of Humanity – Book: An Intimate History of Humanity (Jan. 1996) by Theodore Zeldin.

Anabolic Steroids – some athletes take a form of steroids known as anabolic-androgen steroids or just anabolic steroids to increase their muscle mass and strength.

Analgesic Pain Killer – any member of the group of drugs used to achieve analgesia, relief from pain.

Anemia – blood deficiency.

Anemia Pernicious – an autoimmune disorder in which the body fails to make enough healthy red blood cells (RBCs).

Anemia Iron Deficiency – a condition in which blood lacks adequate healthy red blood cells.

Angiography - or arteriography is a medical imaging technique used to visualize the inside, or lumen, of blood vessels and organs of the body, particularly the arteries, veins, and heart chambers.

Anti-inflammatory – or antiinflammatory refers to the property of a substance or treatment that reduces inflammation or swelling.

Ascites – accumulation of fluid in the peritoneal cavity, causing abdominal swelling.

Attila the Hun – (434–453) the ruler of the Huns until his death. Attila was a leader of the Hunnic Empire. During his reign, he was one of the most feared enemies of the Western and Eastern Roman Empires.

Ayurvedic Herbal Tradition – or Ayurvedic medicine is a system of medicine with historical roots in the Indian subcontinent; a type of alternative medicine.

Bacterial Endocarditis – is an inflammation of the inner tissues of the heart, the endocardium (such as its valves). Caused by infectious agents, or pathogens, which are usually bacterial but other organisms, can also be responsible.

Barbiturates – are drugs that act as central nervous system depressants, and can therefore produce a wide spectrum of effects, from mild sedation to total anesthesia. They are also effective as anxiolytics, hypnotics, and anticonvulsants.

Benzodiazepines – sometimes called benzos, are a class of psychoactive drugs whose core chemical structure is the fusion of a benzene ring and a diazepine ring.

Bilirubin – the yellow breakdown product of normal heme catabolism, caused by the body's clearance of aged red blood cells which contain hemoglobin.

Blood Stasis – or blood stagnation (Xue Yu). Described in TCM theory as a slowing or pooling of the blood due to disruption of Heart Chi.

Blood Tonic – an herbal formula used in Chinese Herbology that will enrich and strengthen the blood.

Bronchopneumonia - inflammation of the lungs, arising in the bronchi or bronchioles.

Candida Albicans – a diploid fungus that grows both as yeast and filamentous cells and a causal agent of opportunistic oral and genital infections.

Candidiasis – a fungal infection; when it affects the mouth, it is called thrush causing white patches on the tongue or other areas of the mouth and throat.

Celiac Sprue – an autoimmune disorder of the small intestine.

Chao – in Chinese Herbology this is a form of dry-frying or cooking herbs prior to use in an herbal prescription.

Chi – the vital energy that flows throughout the body.

Chi Kung – a holistic system of coordinated body posture and movement, breathing, and meditation used for health, spirituality, and martial arts training.

Chi Tonic – a Chinese herbal formula used to strengthen the body's vital energy.

Chinese Herbology – the theory of traditional Chinese herbal therapy, which accounts for the majority of treatments in traditional Chinese medicine (TCM).

Chlordiazepoxide – the discovery of the drug chlordiazepoxide and other benzodiazepines were initially accepted with widespread public approval but were followed with widespread public disapproval.

Cholangiocarcinoma – a form of cancer that is composed of mutated epithelial cells (or cells showing characteristics of epithelial differentiation) that originate in the bile ducts.

Cirrhosis – a late stage of scarring (fibrosis) of the liver caused by forms of liver diseases and conditions, such as hepatitis and chronic alcohol abuse.

Clears Heat – in Chinese medicine resolves feverish conditions that are caused by inflammation.

Clonazepam – aka Klonopin, a medication used to prevent and treat seizures, panic disorder, and for the movement disorder known as akathisia. A tranquilizer known as a benzodiazepine.

Club Drugs – aka rave drugs, are recreational drugs which are associated with discothèques and dance clubs, parties, and raves. Club drugs are a category of convenience, which includes drugs ranging from entactogens and inhalants to stimulants and psychedelics.

Cocaine – aka benzoylmethylecgonine or coke is a strong stimulant mostly used as a recreational drug. Commonly snorted, inhaled, or injected into the veins. Mental effects may include loss of contact with reality, an intense feeling of happiness, or agitation.

Codeine – aka 3-methylmorphine (a naturally occurring methylated morphine) is an opiate used to treat pain.

Coma – a state of unconsciousness in which a person: cannot be awakened; fails to respond normally to painful stimuli, light, or sound; lacks a normal wake-sleep cycle; and does not initiate voluntary actions.

Compress – a pad of absorbent material used to relieve inflammation and swelling.

Congenital Syphilis – present in utero and at birth; occurs when a child is born to a mother with syphilis.

Consumption – or TB (tubercle bacillus), aka phthisis, phthisis pulmonalis, or consumption a widespread, infectious disease caused by various strains of mycobacteria, usually mycobacterium tuberculosis.

Crack-house – a building where drug dealers and drug users buy, sell, produce, and use illegal drugs, including, but not limited to, crack cocaine.

Crohn's Disease – a type of inflammatory bowel disease (IBD) that may affect any part of the gastrointestinal tract from mouth to anus.

Cultural Revolution – the Great Proletarian Cultural Revolution was a social-political movement in the People's Republic of China that was set into motion by Mao Tse Tung, then Chairman of the Communist Party of China.

Cupping – used in Chinese medicine; suction is created on the skin to mobilize blood flow and promote healing.

Dampness – in Chinese medicine this is any kind of turbidity (mucus, phlegm, water, etc.).

Decoction – in Chinese Herbology this is an herbal tea.

Deep Vein Thrombosis – the formation of a blood clot (thrombus) within a deep vein, predominantly in the legs. Pulmonary embolism, a potentially life-threatening complication, is caused by the detachment (embolization) of a clot that travels to the lungs.

Delirium Tremens – caused by withdrawal from alcohol. Physical effects may include shakings, shivering, an irregular heart rate, and sweating.

Dementia – a broad category of brain diseases that cause a long term and often gradual decrease in the ability to think and remember that is great enough to affect a person's daily functioning.

Depressants – a drug that lowers neurotransmission levels, which is to depress or reduce arousal or stimulation, in various areas of the brain. Depressants are also occasionally referred to as downers.

Depression – a state of low mood and aversion to activity that can affect a person's thoughts, behavior, feelings and sense of well-being. People with depressed mood can feel sad, anxious, hopeless, worthless, or restless.

Diabetes Mellitus – a group of metabolic diseases in which there are high blood sugar levels over a prolonged period.

Diarrhea – the condition of having at least three loose or liquid bowel movements each day. Often lasts for a few days and can result in dehydration due to fluid loss.

Diastolic – the diastolic blood pressure number or the bottom number indicates the pressure in the arteries when the heart rests between beats. A normal diastolic blood pressure number is less than eighty.

Diazepam – aka Valium, a medication of the benzodiazepine family that alters the function of the brain to produce a calming effect.

Disturbed Shen – in TCM this is a mental/spiritual imbalance.

Diverticular Disease – occurs when pouches (diverticula) in the intestine, usually the large intestine or colon, become inflamed.

Echocardiography – the use of ultrasound waves to investigate the action of the heart.

Ecstasy – MDMA (methylenedioxy-methamphetamine), popularly known as ecstasy or, more recently, as Molly, is a synthetic, psychoactive drug that has similarities to both the stimulant amphetamine and the hallucinogen mescaline.

Eighteen Buddha Hand – a set of Chi Kung exercises.

Erythematosus – an inflammatory connective tissue disease that is often held to be an autoimmune disease and that occurs chiefly in women, is characterized especially by fever, skin rash, and arthritis, often by acute hemolytic anemia, by small hemorrhages in the skin and mucous membranes, by inflammation of the pericardium, and in serious cases by involvement of the kidneys and central nervous system.

Esophageal Varices – abnormal, enlarged veins in the lower part of the esophagus.

Fatty Liver – aka fatty liver disease (FLD), wherein large vacuoles of triglyceride fat accumulate in liver cells via the process of steatosis (i.e., abnormal retention of lipids within a cell). Despite having multiple causes, fatty liver in those with excessive alcohol intake.

Five–Needle-Auricular-Acupuncture Protocol – used around the world to help people deal with and recover from substance abuse. This protocol has been shown in a variety of clinical settings to be beneficial in the process of detoxification from substance abuse as well as to help with the emotional, physical and psychological attributes involved in addictions.

Gastritis – inflammation of the lining of the stomach.

GHB – Gamma hydroxybutyrate (GHB) aka Gamma-OH – a drug used illicitly for recreational purposes and for date rape. GBH is a central nervous system depressant.

Gonococcal Pharyngitis – an infection of the throat involving the tonsils and the larynx (pharynx), caused by the bacterium Neisseria gonorrhoeae; it is an STD.

Gonorrhea – bacterial infection transmitted by sexual contact. Gonorrhea is caused by the Neisseria gonorrhoeae bacteria.

Goosebumps – goose pimples or goose flesh, the medical term cutis anserina or horripilation, are the bumps on a person's skin at the base of body hairs which may involuntarily develop when a person is cold or experiences strong emotions such as fear, nostalgia, pleasure, euphoria, awe, admiration, and sexual arousal.

Great Leap Forward – made by the Communist Party of China under the leadership of Mao Tse Tung (also known as Mao Zedong) to transform China into a society capable of competing with other industrialized nations, within a short time period.

Hallucinogens – drugs that cause hallucinations (profound distortions in a person's perceptions of reality).

Hangover – the disagreeable physical aftereffects of drunkenness, such as a headache or stomach disorder, usually felt several hours after cessation of drinking.

Harmonize the Center – in Chinese medicine this term refers to settling the stomach.

Hashish – an extract of the cannabis plant, containing concentrations of the psychoactive resins.

Heartburn – a burning sensation in the chest that can extend to the neck, throat, and face; worsened by bending or lying down. The primary symptom of gastroesophageal reflux, which is the movement of stomach acid into the esophagus. On rare occasions, it is due to gastritis (stomach lining inflammation).

Hemolytic Jaundice – jaundice resulting from increased production of bilirubin from hemoglobin as a result of any process (toxic, genetic, or immune) causing increased destruction of erythrocytes.

Hepatitis B – a severe form of viral hepatitis transmitted in infected blood, causing fever, debility, and jaundice.

Hepatitis C – an infection caused by a virus that attacks the liver and leads to inflammation.

Hepatocellular – pertaining to or affecting liver cells.

Hepatoma – cancer originating in the liver, in liver cells. More often called hepatocarcinoma or hepatocellular carcinoma.

Heroin – aka H, smack, boy, horse, brown, black, tar, and others is an opioid analgesic originally synthesized by C. R. Alder Wright in 1874 by adding two acetyl groups to the molecule morphine, which is found naturally in the opium poppy.

Herpes Labiales – fever blisters or cold sores caused by herpes simplex virus type 1. The virus lies latent (dormant) in the body and is reawakened (reactivated) by factors such as stress, sunburn, or fever from a wide range of infectious diseases including colds.

Herpes Simplex Virus (Herpesvirus Hominis, type 2) – member of the herpesvirus family, HSV-2 (which produces most genital herpes) are ubiquitous and contagious. Herpes simplex can be spread through contact with saliva, such as sharing drinks.

Herpes/Genital Herpes – Genital herpes is a common sexually transmitted infection that affects men and women. Features of genital herpes include pain, itching and sores in the genital area.

Holism – in philosophy the theory that parts of a whole are in intimate interconnection, such that they cannot exist independently of the whole, or cannot be understood without reference to the whole, which is thus regarded as greater than the sum of its parts. Holism is often applied to mental states, language, and ecology. In medicine the treating of the whole person, taking into account mental and social factors, rather than just the physical symptoms of a disease.

Hypertension – High blood pressure, defined as a repeatedly elevated blood pressure exceeding 140 over 90 mmHg.

Infection, Abscess and Ulcers – symptoms include redness, pain, warmth, and swelling. They are usually caused by a bacterial infection; often many different types of bacteria are involved in a single infection.

Infertility – diminished or absent ability to conceive and bear offspring. Infertility can have many causes and may be related to factors in the male, female, or both.

Inherited Neuropathies – a group of inherited disorders affecting the peripheral nervous system.

Insomnia – a persistent disorder that can make it hard to fall asleep, hard to stay asleep or both, despite the opportunity for adequate sleep.

Insulin Dependent Type 1 – a form of diabetes mellitus that results from the autoimmune destruction of the insulin-producing beta cells in the pancreas.

Irritable Bowel Syndrome – affects the large intestine (colon). Irritable bowel syndrome commonly causes cramping, abdominal pain, bloating, gas, diarrhea and constipation.

Jaundice – a medical condition with yellowing of the skin or whites of the eyes, arising from excess of the pigment bilirubin and typically caused by obstruction of the bile duct, by liver disease, or by excessive breakdown of red blood cells.

Ketamine – a synthetic compound used as an anesthetic and analgesic drug and also (illicitly) as a hallucinogen.

Kyoshi – This martial art's ranking/title is bestowed upon a Sixth, Seventh of Eighth Degree Black Belt, who is considered an accomplished teacher, and has practiced martial arts for at least twenty-five to thirty years.

Land of Nod – to nod out; to fall asleep, especially when using drugs.

Land of the Dragon - the dragon has long been the symbol of the Emperor of China. As a reference to their ethnic dignity, the people of China often refer to themselves as descendants of the dragon.

Leukemia – cancer that usually begins in the bone marrow and results in high numbers of abnormal white blood cells. These white blood cells are not fully developed and are called blasts or leukemia cells.

Lincoln Detox Program – founded in the South Bronx by political and social activists involved with the Young Lords, including but not limited to the Black Panther Party, the Republic of New Afrika, and Students for a Democratic Society. The clinic offered drug rehabilitation with a holistic approach, employing the use of Chinese Herbology and acupuncture, political education classes and community service.

Liver Cancer – malignant hepatoma is the most common type of liver cancer. Most cases are secondary to either a viral hepatitis infection (hepatitis B or C) or cirrhosis (alcoholism being the most common cause of liver cirrhosis).

Lobar Pneumonia – a form of pneumonia that affects a large and continuous area of the lobe of a lung.

Lorazepam – aka Ativan, a benzodiazepine medication used to treat anxiety disorders. Lorazepam reduces anxiety, interferes with new memory formation, reduces agitation, induces sleep, treats seizures, treats nausea and vomiting, and relaxes muscles.

LSD – a mind altering drug first synthesized by Albert Hofmann in 1938 from ergotamine, a chemical derived by Arthur Stoll from ergot, a grain fungus that typically grows on rye.

Lymphomas – any of a group of blood cell tumors that develop from lymphatic cells. The name often refers to just the cancerous ones rather than all such tumors. Symptoms may include enlarged lymph nodes, fever, drenching sweats, weight loss, itching, and feeling tired.

Malignant Tumors – a tumor that invades surrounding tissues, usually capable of producing metastases, may recur after attempted removal, and is likely to cause death unless adequately treated.

Malnutrition – lack of proper nutrition, caused by not having enough to eat, not eating enough of the right things, or being unable to use the food that one does eat.

Mao Tse Tong – 1893–1976, Chinese Communist leader, chairman of the People's Republic of China 1949–59; chairman of the Chinese Communist Party 1943–76.

Marijuana – Cannabis, also known as marijuana and by numerous other names, a preparation of the Cannabis plant intended for use as a psychoactive drug or medicine.

Massage Therapy – used in Chinese medicine to reduce injuries by improving circulation and lymphatic flow.

Meditation – used in Chinese medicine to improve health; the form of meditation is either standing, sitting or moving meditation which is more commonly known as Tai Chi Chuan or Chi Kung.

Meningitis – a disease caused by the inflammation of the protective membranes covering the brain and spinal cord known as the meninges.

Methadone – used as a pain reliever and as part of drug addiction detoxification and maintenance programs.

Methamphetamine – also called meth, crystal, chalk, and ice, among other terms is an extremely addictive stimulant drug that is chemically similar to amphetamine.

Methylphenidate – a central nervous system (CNS) stimulant of the phenethylamine and piperidine classes used in the treatment of attention deficit hyperactivity disorder (ADHD) and narcolepsy.

Micro-Cosmic Orbit – circulating the Chi (sexual energy) through the small heavenly cycle.

Mind-Altering Narcotic – a chemical substance that changes brain function and results in alterations in perception, mood, or consciousness. These substances may be used recreationally, to purposefully alter one's consciousness, or as entheogens, for ritual, spiritual, or shamanic purposes, as a tool for studying or augmenting the mind.

Moniliasis – infection by fungi of the genus Candida, generally C. Albicans, involving the skin, oral mucosa (thrush), respiratory tract, or vagina; occasionally there is a systemic infection or endocarditis. Aka candidiasis.

Mononucleosis Infectious – or Mono – an infection usually caused by the Epstein-Barr Virus. The virus spreads through saliva, which is why it's sometimes called kissing disease.

Morphine – a pain medication of the opiate type. Acts directly on the central nervous system (CNS) to decrease the feeling of pain.

Moving Meditation – like Tai Chi; Chi Kung a form of moving meditation that uses rhythmic physical movements to focus and center the mind. Chi Kung is also used to regulate, maintain, and heal the body's Chi or energy force.

Moxabustion – in Chinese Herbology this is heat therapy using the herb mugwort.

Mycobacterium Tuberculosis Bacterium – primarily a pathogen of the mammalian respiratory system, it infects the lungs.

Narcotic Painkillers – aka opioid pain relievers used for pain that is severe and is not helped by other types of painkillers. Narcotics work by binding to receptors in the brain, which blocks the feeling of pain.

Narcotic – a chemical agent that induces stupor, coma, or insensibility to pain (also called narcotic analgesic).

Nausea – a sensation of unease and discomfort in the upper stomach with an involuntary urge to vomit. It occasionally precedes vomiting.

Neisseria Gonorrhoeae Bacterium – a species of gram-negative coffee bean-shaped diplococci bacteria responsible for the sexually transmitted infection gonorrhea.

Neolithic Period – the period of human culture that began around ten-thousand years ago in the Middle East. Characterized by the beginning of farming, the domestication of animals, and the development of crafts such as pottery and weaving, and the making of polished stone tools.

Neuropathy – the disease or dysfunction of one or more peripheral nerves, typically causing numbness or weakness.

Non-Insulin Dependent Type 2 – relating to or denoting a type of diabetes in which there is some insulin secretion. Such diabetes typically develops in adulthood and can frequently be managed by diet and hypoglycemic agents.

Nuyorican – a Puerto Rican living in the U.S., especially in New York City.

Obamacare – a federal law providing for a fundamental reform of the U.S. healthcare and health insurance system, signed by President Barack Obama in 2010: formally called Affordable Care Act or Patient Protection and Affordable Care Act.

Opioids – an opium-like compound that binds to one or more of the three opioid receptors of the body.

Opium – a reddish-brown heavy-scented addictive drug prepared from the juice of the opium poppy, used as a narcotic and in medicine as an analgesic.

Opium Den – an establishment where opium is sold and smoked. Patrons recline in order to hold the long opium pipes over oil lamps that heat the drug until it vaporizes and the smoker will inhale the intoxicating vapors.

Overdose – drug overdose or OD describes the ingestion or application of a drug or other substance in quantities greater than are recommended or generally practiced. An overdose may result in a toxic state or death.

Over-the-Counter-Drugs – medicines sold directly to a consumer without a prescription, from a healthcare professional, as compared to prescription drugs, which may be sold only to consumers possessing a valid prescription.

Oxycodone – the active ingredient in OxyContin. Oxycodone is an opioid, a close relative of morphine, heroin, codeine, fentanyl, and methadone.

Painkilling Drugs – (analgesic) used to achieve analgesia, relief from pain. Analgesic drugs act in various ways on the peripheral and central nervous systems. They are distinct from anesthetics, which reversibly eliminate sensation.

Pancreatitis – inflammation of the pancreas. Of the many causes of pancreatitis, the most common are alcohol consumption and gallstones.

Peptic Ulcer – a lesion in the lining (mucosa) of the digestive tract, typically in the stomach or duodenum, caused by the digestive action of pepsin and stomach acid.

Periaperitis Nodosa – aka panarteritis nodosa, Kussmaul disease, Kussmaul-Maier disease or PAN, is a systemic vasculitis of muscular arteries, typically involving renal and visceral vessels but sparing the pulmonary circulation.

Peritonitis – inflammation of the peritoneum, typically caused by bacterial infection either via the blood or after rupture of an abdominal organ.

Pernicious Anemia – a deficiency in the production of red blood cells through a lack of vitamin B12.

Peroneal Muscular Atrophy – a hereditary form of muscular atrophy characterized by progressive wasting of the distal muscles of the extremities, usually affecting the legs before the arms.

Phencyclidine PCP – a street drug known as angel dust that causes physiological changes to the nervous and circulatory system, disturbances in thinking and behavior, and can cause hallucinations, psychotic disorder, mood disorder, and anxiety disorder.

Phenobarbital – a barbiturate, nonselective central nervous system depressant which is primarily used as a sedative hypnotic and also as an anticonvulsant in sub-hypnotic doses.

Phlebitis – inflammation of the walls of a vein.

Pleural Effusion – a buildup of fluid in the pleural space, an area between the layers of tissue that line the lungs and the chest cavity. May also be referred to as effusion or pulmonary effusion.

Pleurisy – inflammation of the pleurae, which impairs their lubricating function and causes pain when breathing. Caused by pneumonia and other diseases of the chest or abdomen.

Pneumonia – lung inflammation caused by bacterial or viral infection, in which the air sacs fill with pus and may become solid. Inflammation may affect both lungs (double pneumonia), one lung (single pneumonia), or only certain lobes (lobar pneumonia).

Portal Hypertension – hypertension (high blood pressure) in the portal vein system, which is composed of the portal vein, and its branches and tributaries. Portal hypertension is defined as elevation of hepatic venous pressure.

Primordial Physicians – ancient healers; shamans, witch doctors, sages, lamas and medicine men.

Pulmonary Tuberculosis – an infectious bacterial disease characterized by the growth of nodules (tubercles) in the tissues, especially the lungs.

Qigong (Chi Kung) – a Chinese system of physical exercises and breath control related to Tai Chi.

Rheumatoid Arthritis – a chronic progressive disease causing inflammation in the joints and resulting in painful deformity and immobility, especially in the fingers, wrists, feet, and ankles.

Robert O'Brien – co-author of the book The Encyclopedia of Alcoholism.

Rohypnol (roofies) – a potent sedative drug of the benzodiazepine class.

Rosicrucian Philosophies – a philosophical secret society founded in late medieval Germany by Christian Rosenkreuz. Doctrine or theology built on esoteric truths of the ancient past, which, concealed from the average man, provide insight into nature, the physical universe and the spiritual realm.

Secobarbital (Seconal) – a barbiturate derivative drug that was patented in 1934 in the U.S. It possesses anesthetic, anticonvulsant, anxiolytic, sedative, and hypnotic properties.

Serum hepatitis – is a liver disease caused by the hepatitis B virus (HBV). The virus can cause lifelong infection, cirrhosis (scarring) of the liver, liver cancer, liver failure and death.

Sexual Dysfunction – (or sexual malfunction or sexual disorder) difficulty experienced by an individual or a couple during any stage of a normal sexual activity, including physical pleasure, desire, preference, arousal or orgasm.

Small Heavenly Cycle – controlling your body's energy and circulating the chi through the micro-cosmic orbit.

Snorting Drugs – the most common way to consume powdered cocaine or certain other drugs. To snort coke means to suck it up your nose, with a straw or rolled up money/paper.

"Sugar" – Diabetes mellitus (aka sugar diabetes)-- a condition that occurs when the body can't use glucose (a type of sugar) normally.

Syphilis – a sexually transmitted infection caused by the spirochete bacterium Treponema pallidum subspecies pallidum. The primary route of transmission is through sexual contact; may also be transmitted from mother to fetus during pregnancy or at birth.

Systemic Lupus – or erythematosus (SLE) – an autoimmune disease in which the body's immune system mistakenly attacks healthy tissue.

Systolic – the blood pressure when the heart is contracting. Specifically the maximum arterial pressure during contraction of the left ventricle of the heart. The time at which ventricular contraction occurs is called systole.

Tai Chi Chuan – moving meditation; a Chinese martial art and system of calisthenics, consisting of sequences of very slow controlled movements.

Tang – a decocted tea or soup in Chinese Herbology.

Taoist Philosophies – a philosophical, ethical, health or religious tradition of Chinese origin, or faith of Chinese exemplification, that emphasizes living in harmony with the Tao.

The Encyclopedia of Alcoholism – Book, examines the history of alcohol and alcoholism, providing detailed information about alcohol abuse.

The National Acupuncture Detoxification Association – a not-for-profit advocacy organization that encourages community wellness through the use of a standardized auricular acupuncture protocol for behavioral health, including addictions, and mental health.

The Shakes – jitteriness followed by a long night of drinking which usually will only stop with more drinking.

The Young Lord's Party – a political active group aka Young Lords Organization in New York (notably Spanish Harlem and the Lower Eastside of Manhattan). A Puerto Rican nationalist group in several U.S. cities, primarily New York City and Chicago.

Theodore Zeldin – a historian and philosopher.

Thrombophlebitis – inflammation of the wall of a vein with associated thrombosis, often occurring in the legs during pregnancy.

Thrombosis – local coagulation or clotting of the blood in a part of the circulatory system.

Thrush – aka oral candidiasis, a condition in which the fungus Candida Albicans accumulates on the lining of the mouth.

Tonics – Chinese herbal elixirs that strengthen and energize the user.

Traditional Chinese Medicine – an ancient medical system aka TCM that provides primary health care; including acupuncture, Chinese herbal medicine, massage (tui na), exercise and breathing therapy (such as Chi kung), and diet and lifestyle advice.

Tranquilizers – drugs used to reduce anxiety, fear, tension, agitation, and related states of mental disturbance.

Tuberculosis – an infectious bacterial disease characterized by the growth of nodules (tubercles) in the tissues, especially the lungs.

Tui Na – a form of Chinese manipulative therapy often used in conjunction with acupuncture, moxabustion, fire cupping, Chinese herbalism, Tai Chi, and Chi Kung.

Ulcerated Nose Lining – sore, ulcer, or a skin lesion; a small furuncle or a boil, an ulcer or simply a crack in inner nasal lining. Pain, redness, inflammation and swelling are the cardinal features of nasal sores.

Ulcerative Colitis – UC; a disease that causes inflammation and sores, called ulcers, in the lining of the rectum and colon. The most common symptoms are pain in the abdomen and blood or pus in diarrhea.

Vomiting – the timing of vomiting can indicate the cause. When appearing shortly after a meal, nausea or vomiting may be caused by food poisoning, gastritis, an ulcer, or bulimia. Nausea or vomiting one to eight hours after a meal may also indicate food poisoning.

Wan – Chinese herbal pills or capsules.

Wei Chi – in traditional Chinese medicine this is the immune system.

Wing Chun – a Chinese Martial Art from Canton Province, China. As Bruce Lee's original martial style, now one of the most popular forms of Chinese Kung Fu practiced today.

Withdrawal – the discontinuance of administration or use of a drug; the syndrome of often painful physical and psychological symptoms that follows discontinuance of an addicting drug.

Withdrawal Syndrome – also called a discontinuation syndrome is a set of symptoms occurring in discontinuation or dosage reduction of some types of medications. The risk of a discontinuation syndrome occurring increases with dosage and length of use.

Yin & Yang – in Chinese philosophy, medicine and religion there are two principles, one negative, dark, and feminine (yin) and one positive, bright, and masculine (yang) whose interaction influences the destinies of creatures and things.

Appendix Section III

Cross-Reference Table of Herbs

Chinese Herb	Botanical/Zoological Name	Common Name
Ai Ye 艾葉	*Artemisia Argyi*	Argy Wormwood Leaf
Ba Ji Tian 巴戟天	*Morinda Officinalis*	Morinda Root
Bai Dou Kou 白豆蔻	*Amomim Kravanh*	Cardamom
Bai Ji 白芨	*Bletilla Striata*	Hyacinth Bletilla Tuber
Bai Qian 白前	*Cynanchum Stauntoni*	Cynanchum Rhizome
Bai Shao 白芍	*Paeonia Lactiflora*	White Peony Root
Bai Zhu 白朮	*Atractylodes Macrocephala*	White Atractylodes
Bai Zi Ren 柏子仁	*Platycladus Orientalis*	Biota Seeds
Ban Xia 半夏	*Pinellia Ternata*	Half Summer
Bei Mu 川貝	*Bulbus Fritillariae*	Fritillaria
Bei Sha Shen 北沙蔘	*Radix Glehniae*	Glehnia
Bie Jia 鱉甲	*Trionyx Sinensis*	Turtle Shell
Bing Lang 檳榔	*Araca Catechu*	Betel Nut
Bing Tang 冰糖	*raw granulated sugar*	Sugar
Bo He 薄荷	*Mentha Haplocalyx*	Mint
Bu Gu Zhi 補骨脂	*Psoralea Corylifolia*	Psoralea Fruit
Cang Zhu 草烏	*Atractylodes Lancea*	Atractylodes Rhizome
Chai Hu 柴胡	*Bupleurum Chinense*	Bupleurum
Che Qian Zi 車前子	*Plantago Asiatica*	Plantago Seed
Chen Pi 陳皮	*Citrus Reticulate*	Tangerine Peel
Chi Shao 赤芍	*Paeonia Veitchii*	Red Peony Root
Chuan Lian Zi 川楝子	*Melia Toosendan*	Sichuan Chinaberry
Chuan Mu Tong 川木通	*Clematis Armandii*	Clematis
Chuan Niu Xi 川牛膝	*Cyathula Officinalis*	Cyathula Root
Chuan Xiong 川芎	*Ligusticum Chuanxiong*	Cnidium
Da Fu Zi 檳榔	*Areca Catechu*	Betel Nut Peel
Da Huang 大黃	*Rheum Palmatum*	Rhubarb Root

Chinese Herb	Botanical/Zoological Name	Common Name
Da Ji 大蓟	*Euphorbia Pekinensis*	Knoxia
Da Zao 大棗	*Ziziphus Jujuba*	Jujube
Dan Dou Chi 淡豆豉	*Semen Sojae Preparatum*	Prepared Soybean
Dan Shen 丹參	*Salvia Miltiorrhiza*	Salvia Root
Dan Zhu Ye 淡竹葉	*Lophatherum Gracile*	Bland Bamboo Leaves
Dang Gui 當歸	*Angelica Sinensis*	Chinese Angelica
Dang Shen 党參	*Codonoposis Pilosula*	Codonopsis
Di Gu Pi 地骨皮	*Lycium Barbarum*	Wolfberry Root Bark
Du Zhong 杜仲	*Eucommia Ulmoides*	Eucommia Bark
E Jiao 阿胶	*Equus Asinus*	Ass-Hide Glue
Fang Feng 防風	*Ledebouriellae Radix*	Siler
Feng Mi 蜂蜜	*Apis Cerana*	Honey
Fu Ling 茯苓	*Poria Cocos*	Tuckahoe
Fu Shen 茯神	*Poriae*	Hoelen Center
Fu Xiao Mai 浮小麦	*Triticum Aestivum*	Wheat Levis
Fu Zi 附子	*Aconditum Carmichaeli*	Aconite
Gan Cao 甘草	*Glycyrrhiza Uralensis*	Licorice Root
Gan Jiang 乾薑	*Zingiber Officinale*	Ginger, Dried
Gan Jiang Chao 干姜	*Zingiberis Officinale*	Dried Ginger Cooked
Gan Qi 幹漆	*Toxiodendron Vernicifluum*	Dried Lacquer
Gan Sui 甘遂	*Euphorbia Kansui*	Gansui Root
Ge Gen 葛根	*Radix Puerariae*	Kudzu
Ge Hua 葛花	*Flos Puerariae*	Kudzu Flower
Gou Qi Zi 枸杞子	*Lycii Fructus*	Wolfberry
Gou Teng 勾藤	*Uncaria Rhynchophylla*	Gambir
Gui Zhi 桂枝	*Cinnamomum Cassia*	Cinnamon Twigs
Hai Piao Xiao 乌贼骨	*Sepiaella Maindroni*	Cuttlefish Bone
He Shou Wu 何首乌	*Polygonum Multiflorum*	Polygonum

Chinese Herb	Botanical/Zoological Name	Common Name
He Zi 诃子	*Terminalia Chebula*	Terminalia Fruit
Hong Hua 紅花	*Carthamus Tinctorius*	Carthamus
Hong Teng 大血藤	*Sargentodoxa Cuncata*	Sargentodoxa Vine
Hou Po 厚朴	*Magnolia Officinalis*	Magnolia Bark
Hua Jiao 花椒	*Zanthoxylum Bungeanum*	Prickly Ash Pepper
Huang Bai 黄柏	*Phellodendrom Amurense*	Cork Tree Bark
Huang Jing 黄精	*Rhizoma Polygonati*	Solomon's Seal
Huang Lian 黄連	*Coptis Chinensis*	Coptis Root
Huang Qi 黄芪	*Astragalus Membranaceus*	Mongolian Milkvetch
Huang Qin 黄芩	*Schutellaria Baicalensis*	Baikal Skullcap Root
Huo Ma Ren 火麻仁	*Fructus Cannabis*	Hemp Seeds
Huo Xiang 广藿香	*Agastache Vugosus*	Aromatic Bean Leaf
Ji Nei Jin 鸡内金	*Gallus*	Chicken Gizzard
Ji Xue Teng 鸡血藤	*Spatholobus Suberectus*	Spatholobus
Jiang Huang 姜黄	*Curcuma Longa*	Turmeric
Jie Geng 桔梗	*Platycodon Grandiflorum*	Platycodon
Jin Yin Hua 金银花	*Lonicera Japonica*	Honeysuckle Flower
Ju Hua 菊花	*Chrysanthemum Morifolium*	Chrysanthemum
Ku Shen 苦参	*Sophora Flavescens*	Sophora Root
Ku Xing Ren 杏仁	*Prunus Armeniaca*	Apricot Seed
Kuan Dong Hua 冬花	*Tussilago Farfara*	Coltsfoot Flowers
La Jiao 辣椒	*Capsicum Annuum*	Cayenne Red Pepper
Lai Fu Zi 莱菔子	*Raphanus Sativus*	Radish Seed
Lao Cong Bai 葱白	*Allium Fistulosum*	Scallion, sliced
Lian Fang 莲房	*Nelumbo Nucifera*	Lotus Leaf Receptacle
Lian Qiao 连翘	*Forsythia Suspensa*	Forsythia
Ling Xiao Hua 凌霄花	*Flos Campsis*	Trumpet Creeper
Long Dan 龙胆	*Gentiana Scabra*	Gentian
Lu Feng Fang 露蜂房	*Nidus Vespae*	Hornet's Nest

Chinese Herb	Botanical/Zoological Name	Common Name
Lu Gen 芦根	*Rhizoma Phragmitis*	Reed Rhizome
Lu Jiao Jiao 鹿角胶	*Cervus Nippon*	Deer Horn Gelatin
Mai Men Dong 麦冬	*Ophiopogon Japonicas*	Lush Winter Wheat
Mai Ya 麦芽	*Hordeum Vulgare*	Barley Sprout
Mang Xiao 芒硝	*Natrii Sulfas*	Sodium Sulfate
Meng Chong 虻蟲	*Tabanus Bivttatus*	Gadfly
Mo Yao 没药	*Commiphora Myrrha*	Myrrh
Mu Dan Pi 牡丹皮	*Paeonia Suffruticosa*	Tree Peony Bark
Mu Li 牡蛎	*Ostrea Gigas*	Oyster Shell
Mu Xiang 木香	*Aucklandiae Lappa*	Costus Root
Pi Pa Ye 枇杷叶	*Eriobotrya Japonica*	Loquat Leaf
Po Xiao 芒硝	*Sal Glauberis*	Sodium Sulfate
Pu Gong Ying 蒲公英	*Taraxacum Mongolicum*	Asian Dandelion
Pu Huang 蒲黃炭	*Typha Angustifolia*	Bulrush
Qi Cao 蛴螬	*Holotrichia Diamphala*	Coleopteran Insect
	(Lachnostema)	Larva (White Grub)
Qian Cao 茜草	*Radix Rubiae*	India Madder Root
Qian Hu 前胡	*Peucedanum Pracruptorum*	Hog-Fennel Root
Qian Niu Zi 牵牛子	*Pharbitis Nil*	Pharbitis Seed
Qiang Huo 羌活	*Notopterygum Incisum*	Notopteygium Root
Qiang Lang 蜣螂	*Catharsium*	Dung Beetle
Qing Fen 轻粉	*Calomelas*	Calomel
Qing Pi 青皮	*Citrus Reticulata, Blanco*	Green Tangerine Peel
Qu Mai 瞿麦	*Dianthus Superbus*	Dianthus
Ren Shen 人参	*Panax Ginseng*	Ginseng
Rou Cong Rong 肉苁蓉	*Cistanche*	Cistanche Salsa
Rou Dou Kou 肉豆蔻	*Myristica Fragrans*	Nutmeg
Rou Gui 肉桂	*Cinnamomum Cassia*	Cinnamon Bark
San Qi 三七	*Panax Notoginseng*	Pseudoginseng

Chinese Herb	Botanical/Zoological Name	Common Name
Sang Bai Pi 桑白皮	*Morus Alba*	Mulberry Bark
Sang Ye 桑叶	*Morus Alba*	Mulberry Leaf
Sha Ren 砂仁	*Amomum Villosum*	Amomum Fruit
Shan Yao 山药	*Dioscorea Opposite*	Yam Rhizome
Shan Zha 山楂	*Crataegus Cuneata*	Hawthorne Fruit
Shan Zhu Yu 山茱萸	*Corni Fructus*	Dogwood Fruit
She Gan 射干	*Belamcanda Chinensis*	Blackberry Lily
She Xiang 麝香	*Moschus Berezovskii*	Musk
Shen Qu 神曲	*Massa Fermentata*	Medicated Leaven
Sheng Di Huang 生地黄	*Rehmannia Glutinosa*	Rehmannia, Dried
Sheng Jiang 生姜	*Zingiber Officinale*	Ginger, Fresh
Sheng Ma 升麻	*Cimicifuga Heracleifolia*	Cimicguga
Shi Chang Pu 石菖蒲	*Rhizome Acori*	Acorus
Shi Gao 生石膏	*Gypsum Fibrosum*	Gypsum
Shi Hu 石斛	*Dendrobium Loddigesii*	Dendrobium Stem
Shi Lian Zi 石莲子	*Sinocrassulae Indicae*	Black Lotus Seed
Shi Wei 石韦	*Pyrosia Sheareri*	Japanese Felt Fern
Shu Di Huang 熟地黄	*Rehmanniae, Preparata*	Rehmannia, Cooked
Shu Fu Chong 鼠妇虫	*Armadillidium Vulgare*	Pillbug, Dried
Shui Zhi 水蛭	*Hirudo Nipponica*	Leech, Dried
Si Gua Luo 丝瓜络	*Luffa Cylindrical*	Luffa Fiber
Suan Zao Ren 酸枣仁	*Ziziphus Jujuba*	Spiny Date Seed
Tao Ren 桃仁	*Prunus Persica*	Peach Seed
Tian Hua Fen 天花粉	*Trichosanthes Kirilowii*	Trichosanthes Root
Tian Kui Zi 天葵子	*Semiaquilegia Adoxoides*	Semiaquileqia
Tian Men Dong 天門冬	*Asparagus Cochinchinensis*	Asparagus Tuber
Tian Nan Xing 天南星	*Arisaema Consanguineum*	Jack In The Pulpit
Ting Li Zi 葶苈子	*Descurainia Sophia*	Lepidum
Tu Bei Chong 土鳖虫	*Eupolyphaga Sinensis*	Eupolyphaga

Chinese Herb	Botanical/Zoological Name	Common Name
Tu Fu Ling 土茯苓	*Smilax Glabra*	Smilax
Tu Si Zi 菟絲子	*Cuscuta Chinensis*	Dodder Seed
Wa Leng Zi 瓦楞子	*Arca Subcrenata*	Ark Shell
Wu Ling Zhi Chao 五灵脂	*Trogopterius Xanthipes*	Pteropus Feces
Wu Mei 乌梅	*Fructus Mume*	Dark Plum fruit
Wu Wei Zi 五味子	*Schisandra Chinensis*	Schizandra
Wu Yao 烏藥	*Lindera Strychnifolia*	Lindera Root
Wu Zhu Yu 吳茱萸	*Evodia Rutaecarpa*	Evodia
Xi Fan Lian 西番莲	*Passiflora Incarnata*	Passionflower
Xiang Fu 香附	*Cyperus Rotundus*	Nutgrass Rhizome
Xiao Hui Xiang 小茴香	*Foeniculum Vulgare*	Fennel Seed
Xuan Shen 玄參	*Scrophularia Ningpoensis*	Figwort Root
Xu Duan 續斷	*Dipsacus Asper*	Himalayan Teasel
Yan Hu Suo 延胡索	*Corydalis Turtschaninovii*	Corydalis
Ye Ju Hua 野菊花	*Chrysanthemum Indicum*	Chrysanthemum
Yi Mu Cao 益母草	*Leonurus Heterophyllus*	Motherwort Herb
Yi Tang 饴糖	*Sacchrum Granorum*	Maltose
Yi Yi Ren 薏苡仁	*Coix Lacryma-Jobi*	Coix Seeds
Yin Chen 茵陈	*Artemisia Scoparia*	Wormwood
Ying Su Ke 罌粟壳	*Pericarpium Papaveris*	Poppy Husk
Yu Zhu 玉竹	*Polygonatum Odoratum*	Solomon's Seal
Yuan Hua 芫花	*Daphne Genkwa*	Lilac Daphne
Yuan Zhi 遠志	*Polyala Tenuifolia*	Siberian Milkwort
Ze Xie 澤瀉	*Alisma Orientalis*	Water Plantain
Zhe Bai Mu 浙貝毋	*Fritillaria Verticillata*	Fritillary Bulb
Zhi Gan Cao 甘草	*Radix Glycyrrhizae*	Licorice
Zhi Ke 枳殼	*Citrus Aurantium*	Bitter Orange Fruit
Zhi Mu 知母	*Anemarrhena Aphodeloides*	Anemarrhena
Zhi Shi 炒枳實	*Citrus Aurantium*	Bitter Orange
Zhi Zi 栀子	*Gardenia Jasminoides*	Gardenia
Zhu Ling 豬苓	*Polyporus Umbellatus*	Polyporus

Zhu Ru 竹茹	*Bambusa Breviflora*	Bamboo Shavings
Zhu Ye 苦竹叶	*Phyllostachys Nigra*	Bamboo Leaves
Zi Hua Di Ding 紫花丁	*Viola Yedoensis*	Tokyo Violet
Zi Su Ye 紫蘇	*Perilla Frutescens*	Perilla Leaf
Zi Wan 紫苑	*Asteris*	Tartarian Aster

Appendix Section IV

Alphabetical List of Herbal Formulas

Appendix Section V
Illnesses Associated With Alcohol and Drug Use

Appendix Section VI

Sources for Herbal Formulas

The following companies specialize in online and mail order sales of herbs and herbal formulas. The first company listed is owned by Thomas Richard Joiner, author of this book. This online-based company not only provides herbal formulas, but also takes great pride in the herbal and martial knowledge we share with our customers.

To purchase Chinese herbs in bulk, patent formulas, or any of the herbal formulas discussed in this book, please contact:

Sea of Chi
Aka: Treasures from the Sea of Chi
200 Montecito Avenue # 304
Oakland, CA 94610
Phone: 510-451-0945, or 800-641-0945
Email: info@seaofchi.com
www.seaofchi.com

To purchase Chinese herbs in bulk or patent formulas:
Mayway Corp.
1338 Mandela Parkway
Oakland, CA 94607
Phone: 800-262-9929
Fax: 800-909-2828
www.mayway.com

NuHerbs Company
3820 Penniman Avenue
Oakland, CA 94619
Phone: 510-534-4372, or 800-233-4307
Fax: 510-534-4384
www.nuherbs.com

Chinese herbal formulas may be purchased from the following retail Chinese herb stores in the USA.

AT Trading
121 Mott Street
New York, NY 10013
Phone: 212-925-8333

New Kam Man
200 Canal St
New York, NY 10013
Phone: 212-571-0330

Ewa Trading Co.
80 Mulberry St
New York, NY 10013
Phone: 212-964-2017

Yin Wall City
2347 S Wentworth Ave
Chicago, IL 60616
Phone: 312-808-1122

Bark Lee Tong
229 W Cermak Rd
Chicago, IL 60686
Phone: 312-225-1988

Far East Center
734 N Broadway
Los Angeles, CA 90012
Phone: 213-617-0020

Universal Family Wellness Clinic
4209 Santa Monica Blvd
Los Angeles, CA 90029
Phone: 323-617-5027

Wing Hop Fung Ginseng
727 N Broadway
Los Angeles, CA 90012
Phone: 213-626-7200

Nam Bac Hong
75 Harrison Ave
Boston, MA 02111
Phone: 617-426-8227

The Ginseng House
6230 SW 8th St
West Miami, FL 33144
Phone: 305-264-7774

Bao An Herbs
705 South King St
Seattle, WA 98104
Phone: 206-227-1619

References

Appendix Section VII
Reference Sources for Herbal Formulas

Bob Flaws,
Hit Medicine Chinese Medicine in Injury Management
(Boulder, Colorado: Blue Poppy Press, 1983)

Dan Bensky and Andrew Gamble,
Chinese Herbal Medicine Materia Medica Revised Edition
(Seattle, Washington: Eastland Press, 1993)

Dan Bensky and Randall Barolet,
Chinese Herbal Medicine Formulas and Strategies
(Eastland Press, 1990)

Daniel P. Reid,
Chinese Herbal Medicine
(Boston, Massachusetts: Shambhala Pub., Inc. 1986)

Jake Fratkin,
Chinese Herbal Patent Medicines
(Boulder, Colorado: Shya Publications, 2001)

James Ramholz,
Shaolin and Taoist Herbal Training Formulas
(Chicago, Illinois: Silk Road, 1992)

Pang, T.Y.
Chinese Herbal: An Introduction
(Honolulu, Hawaii: Tai School of Philosophy and Art, 1982)

Patriarch De Chan,
Shaolin Secret Formulas for the Treatment of External Injury
(Boulder, Colorado: Blue Poppy Press, 1995)